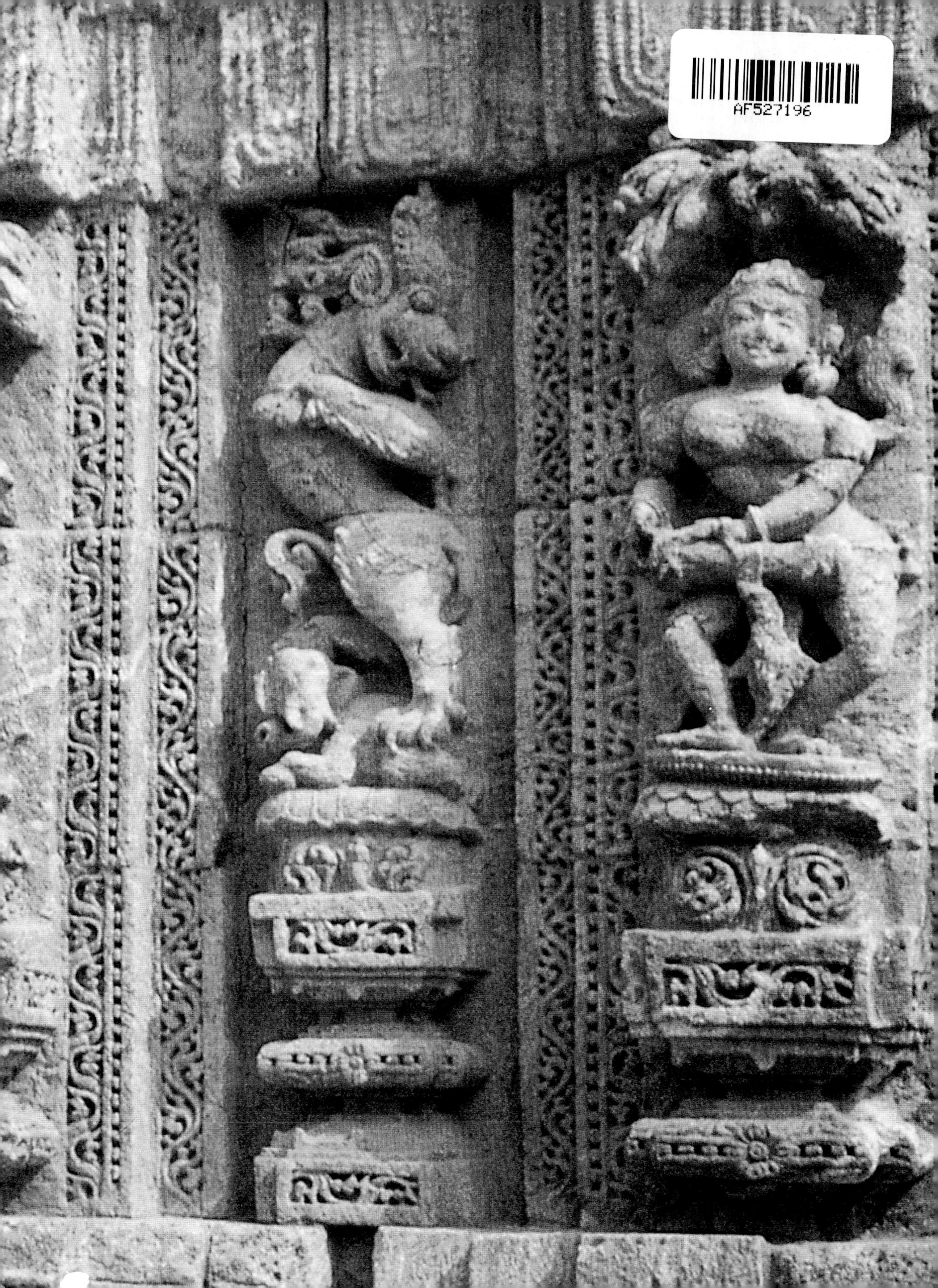

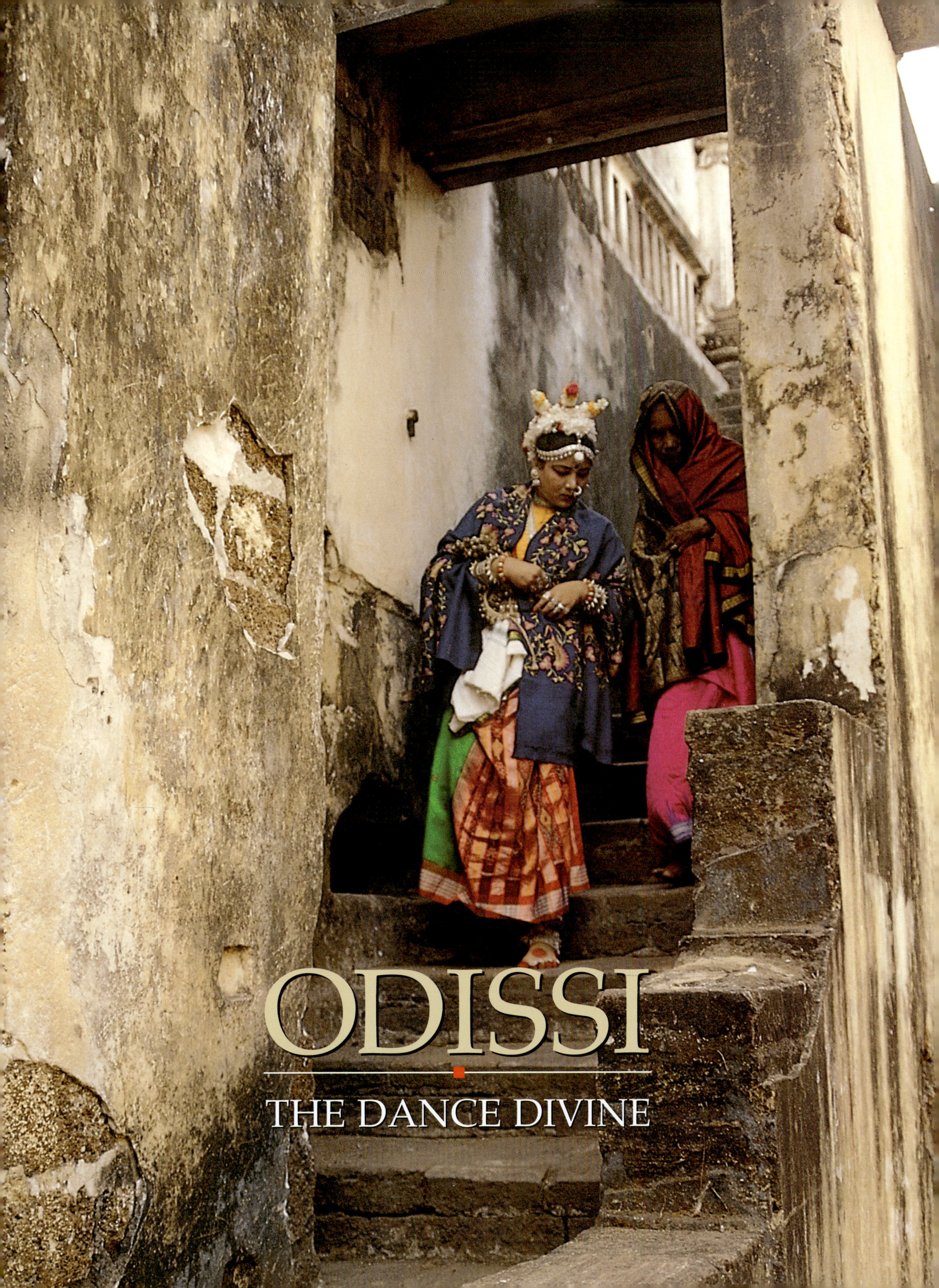

ODISSI

THE DANCE DIVINE

Cover: An Odissi dance performance at the famous Sun Temple, Konark.

ODISSI

THE DANCE DIVINE

Previous page: A contemporary dancer of the mahari *style leading the last living* mahari *Shashimoni of the Jagannath Temple, Puri.*

Following double spread: The magnificent Jagannath Temple, Puri.

ODISSI

THE DANCE DIVINE

RANJANA GAUHAR

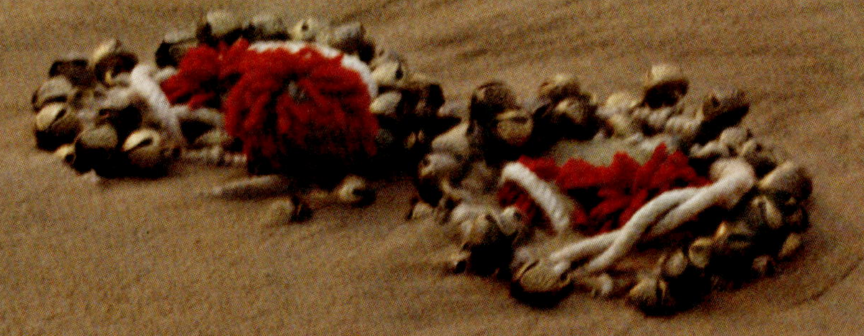

PHOTOGRAPHS BY
DUSHYANT PARASHER

NIYOGI
BOOKS

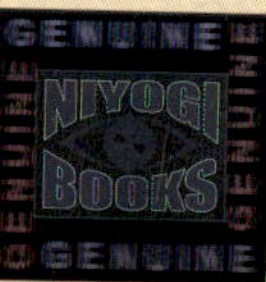

Published by
NIYOGI BOOKS
D-78, Okhla Industrial Area, Phase-I
New Delhi-110 020, INDIA
Tel: 91-11-26816301, 49327000
Fax: 91-11-26810483, 26813830
Email: niyogibooks@gmail.com
Website: www.niyogibooksindia.com

Editor: Alka Raghuvanshi
Design: Dushyant Parasher
ISBN: 81-89738-17-8

Year of Publication: 2007
2nd impression: 2009
3rd impression: 2017

Notice: *Most of the photographs of the gurus and individual artists featured on pages 130 to 141, were provided by the gurus and the artists themselves and their photographers are not known to us. However, we would like to hear from the respective photographers and give them credit for their work, in future editions.*
—Author and Publisher

Printed at: Niyogi Offset Pvt. Ltd., New Delhi, India

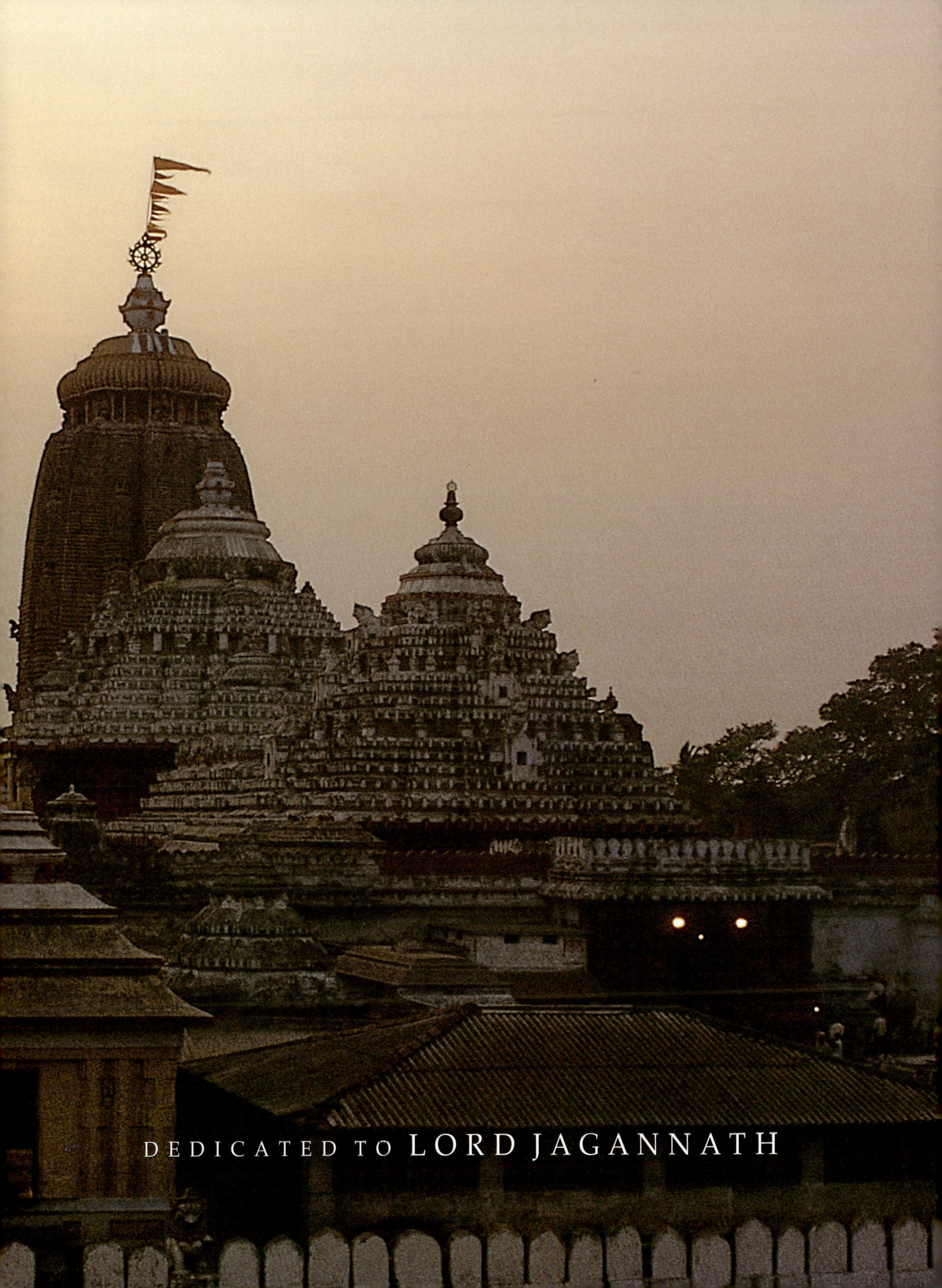

DEDICATED TO LORD JAGANNATH

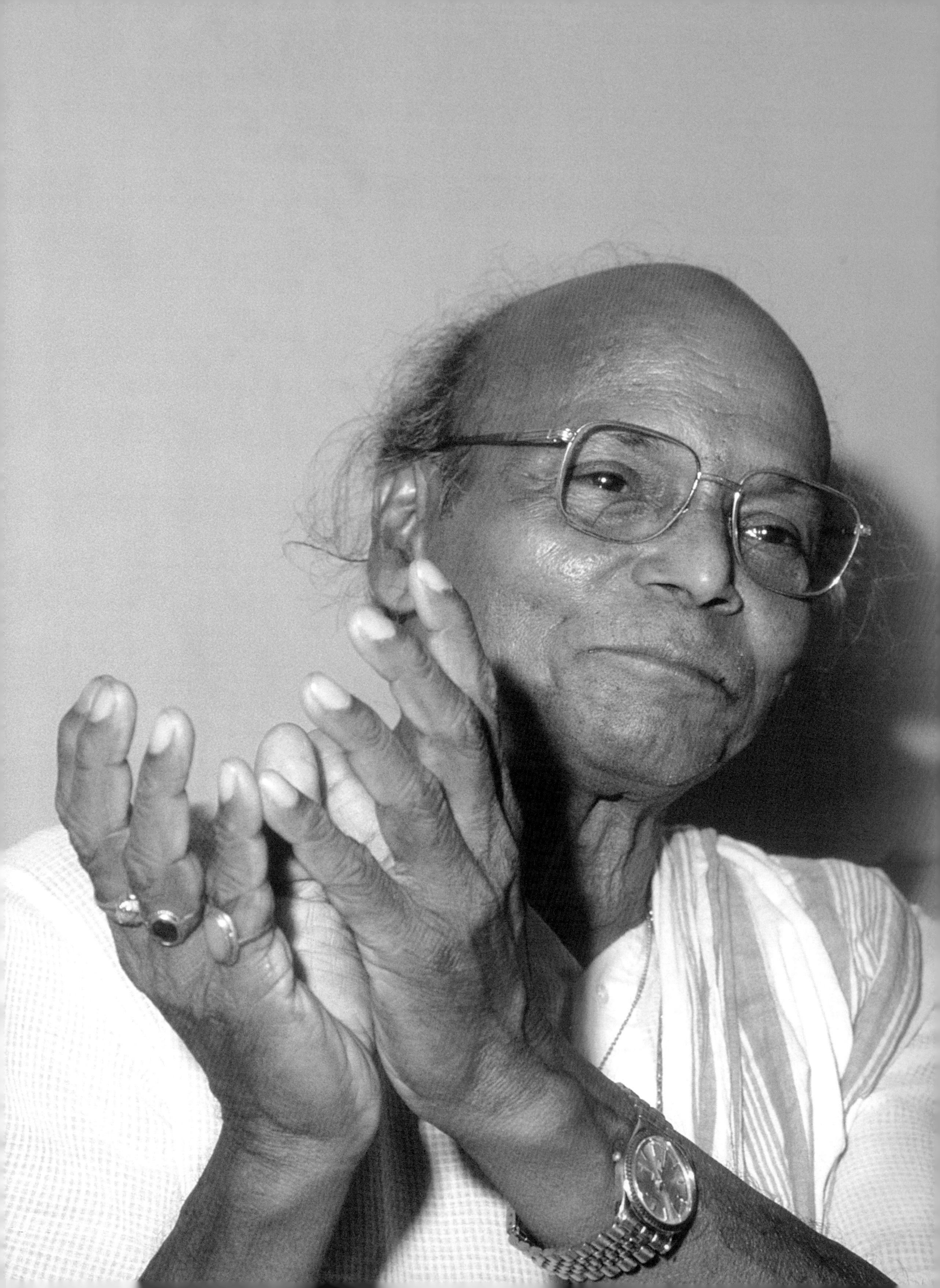

MESSAGE

It gives me great joy to know that you are publishing a book on Odissi, which will certainly serve as a pathfinder to the present and future generations in the field of Indian classical dance.

Words may not be enough to eulogize your dedication to Indian classical heritage and achievements *par excellence;* your versatile accomplishments have helped you deservedly to carve a niche for yourself in the contemporary art and culture scenario.

I will be happy if my good wishes and blessings encourage you to soar to newer heights and contribute in propagating this fascinating form of Indian dance.

Kelucharan Mohapatra
Bhubaneswar

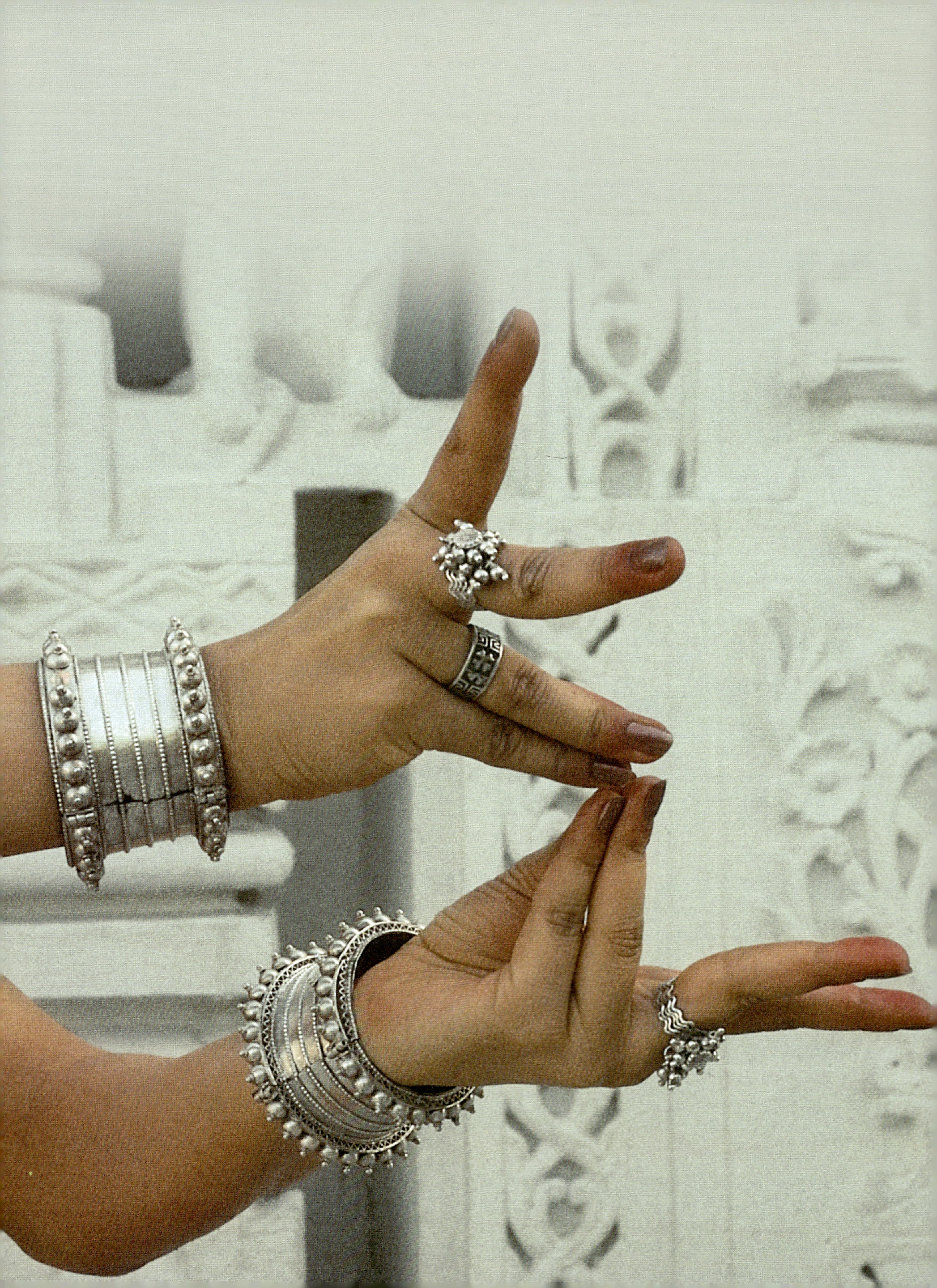

CONTENTS

AUTHOR'S NOTE

As a child, I had always cherished a desire to be like a bird to enjoy the freedom of hopping from tree to tree and soaring into the skies. It must have been a spiritual quest for freedom. I heard music in everything around me and I could sense the rhythms of Nature through my body. My spirit yearned to capture its myriad patterns and translate them into movement. There was an irresistible urge within me to let my restless spirit be in harmony with Nature, to use rhythm to express my soul. I felt I simply had to dance.

A seemingly insignificant incident strengthened my determination to be a dancer. I was in class seven. One day, the teacher chose a few girls of my class to perform in a group dance. I eagerly waited for my name to be called, but in vain. It broke my heart and I resolved to beat them all one day! Today when I look back, I laugh at my naiveté.

Then one day, I saw a dance. It was what my soul and heart had been yearning for—the music and the movements transported me to a land celestial. I was struck by the *apsara*-like look, the scintillating music and the lyrical, sculpturesque rhythm of the dance. I knew instantly that this was the dance I wanted to learn. The next challenge was to find a teacher who could teach me the *apsara* dance, which I later discovered was called Odissi.

One afternoon, when I had nearly lost hope of finding a teacher, a friend excitedly informed me about a person who could teach me. It was none other than Guru Mayadhar Raut. Thus began my quest and never-ending thirst to learn more and more about this fascinating dance.

During the training, which was hard, arduous and tiring yet rejuvenating, nurturing and soothing I felt possessed, as though in a trance. Not once did my enthusiasm and romance for Odissi wane. In the beginning, when I was learning the basic steps, I was fascinated by the way my body had to bend, move and turn to execute the movements. Because the dance was highly stylised, it was very interesting as well as challenging. I could hardly wait to learn a full composition. Listening to the melodious music of Odissi, my heart would swell with emotions and tears would roll down my face. But what moved me most was the spiritual and aesthetic strength of the *Geeta*

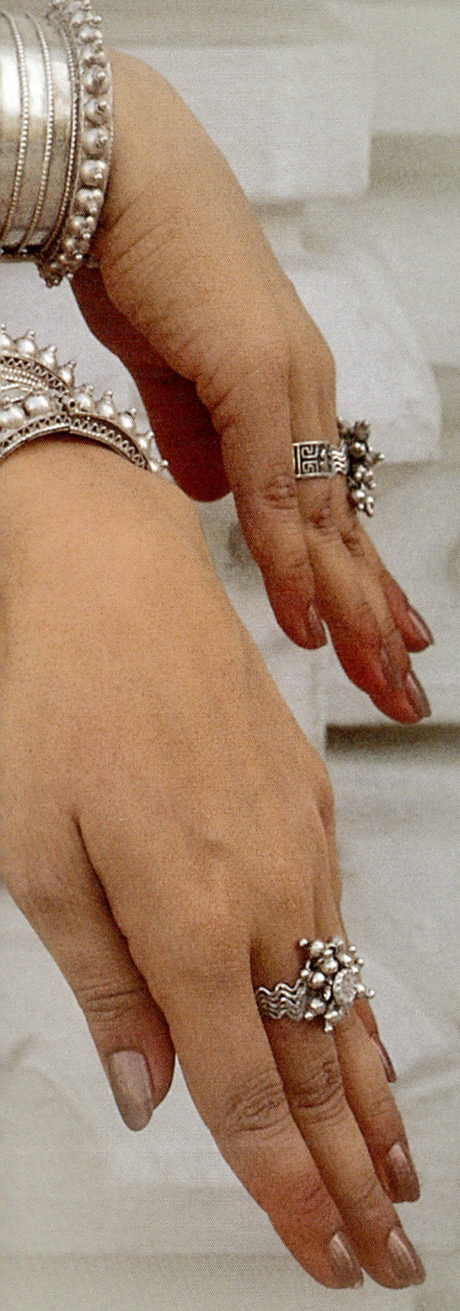

Govinda—its *shringara bhakti,* Radha and Krishna's graceful fulfilment and dignity in love, in union or in separation; the rich sensuality of their romantic expression alongside the serene spirituality in the realisation of their love.

Later, when I learnt the *ashtapadis* from the *Geeta Govinda,* I would imagine Krishna dancing around me—so powerful was the impact of Jayadeva's lyrics that I could transcend from the physical to the metaphysical. And I could visualise Jayadeva's lyrics vividly and relate to Radha's passion and devotion for Odissi is intrinsically passionate in its embrace of womanhood.

When I dance a *pallavi,* my feet love executing the intricate rhythmic patterns and my body sways with the melody of the *raga* like the branches of a tree. I am transported to the divine. No wonder Odissi is called 'the dance of the Gods'.

My search for dance and freedom of spirit led me to Odissi. I found in it serenity, strength and a sense of purpose. With each day, I hungered to learn more. I found my biggest inspiration in the legendary Odissi maestro Guru Kelucharan Mohapatra. I feel blessed to have experienced the splendour of his art and the brilliance of his intellect, and am grateful for the grace he has bestowed on me.

He has given me so much love. I salute his manifold contributions to this dance as the architect of contemporary Odissi, as performer, teacher, choreographer and researcher. Indeed the last fifty years of Odissi may well be called the 'Kelucharan era'. The global awareness and positioning of Odissi can be attributed to none other. Then there are the exponents of the art across the world, the global Odissi family—from whom I derive strength and motivation.

This journey of discovering Odissi has taught me much more than dance and rhythm. I realised that there is something inherent in human nature, and that is the search for the divine. And Odissi is my path to divinity.

Odissi—The Dance Divine is my tribute to my chosen journey—the only factor that has given direction and depth to my life, helped me experience passion, devotion and overwhelming love. It has inspired me to keep going, to fly higher than the highest that I can, and strive to better the best in me. This book comes from my heart and is the culmination of the experience of many years of learning, practising and teaching the dance, and years of travelling to share and convey the fascinating beauty of this art form. In this book, which assimilates the crux of my life, there are many people to thank.

First and foremost, my *Guruji*, Guru Mayadhar Raut, who made me aware of the fine nuances of this form, its historical background and content. He has brought me from the point of my first step, my first movement in dance to where I am today. His Odissi compositions—music and dance choreographies—have always been inspiring. His choreography and visualisation of the *ashtapadis* from the *Geeta Govinda* matched the poetic description of Jayadeva—they move me and motivate me even today. Aloka Paniker, who added *bhava* and *rasa* in the *abhinaya* aspect of the dance to the knowledge imparted to me by *Guruji*. She added substance to my performance by polishing and giving me the correct perception of dance. They both patiently bore my shortcomings and coped with my insatiable desire to learn the dance form.

This book has taken many years of rigorous research, writing and rewriting many drafts, editing and polishing. I thank Debbie Smith, Dr Itishree Sahoo, Sapna Khanna and Tonushree Jaggi, for tirelessly working without flinching from fine-combing the book that 'just one more time'. The guidance and advice by Dr Alka Raghuvanshi has been invaluable.

I thank my parents who are no more, for giving me the freedom of choice—to be an Odissi dancer, an art form with which they were not familiar. I am what I am because of them. I can never really thank them enough for supporting me, for instilling sound values in me, for sensitising me to our fabulous cultural heritage and infusing in me love and devotion for the same—an aspect I have come to regard as one of the highest forms of patriotism.

Finally, and most of all, I thank my son Sidharth, for allowing me the time to continue to love Odissi and its related work, because of which he was understandably deprived of my attention for many hours each day.

Ranjana Gauhar

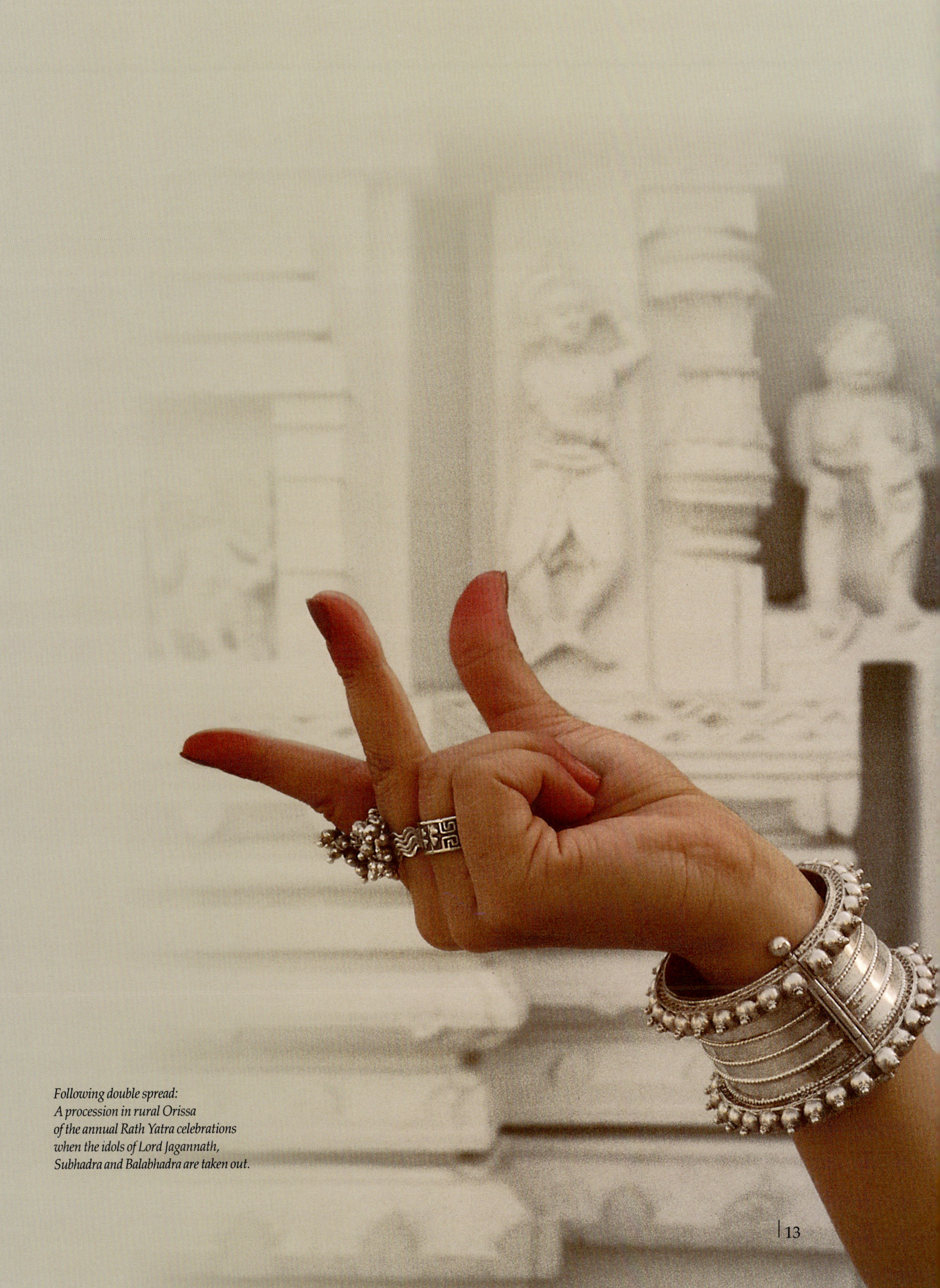

Following double spread:
A procession in rural Orissa of the annual Rath Yatra celebrations when the idols of Lord Jagannath, Subhadra and Balabhadra are taken out.

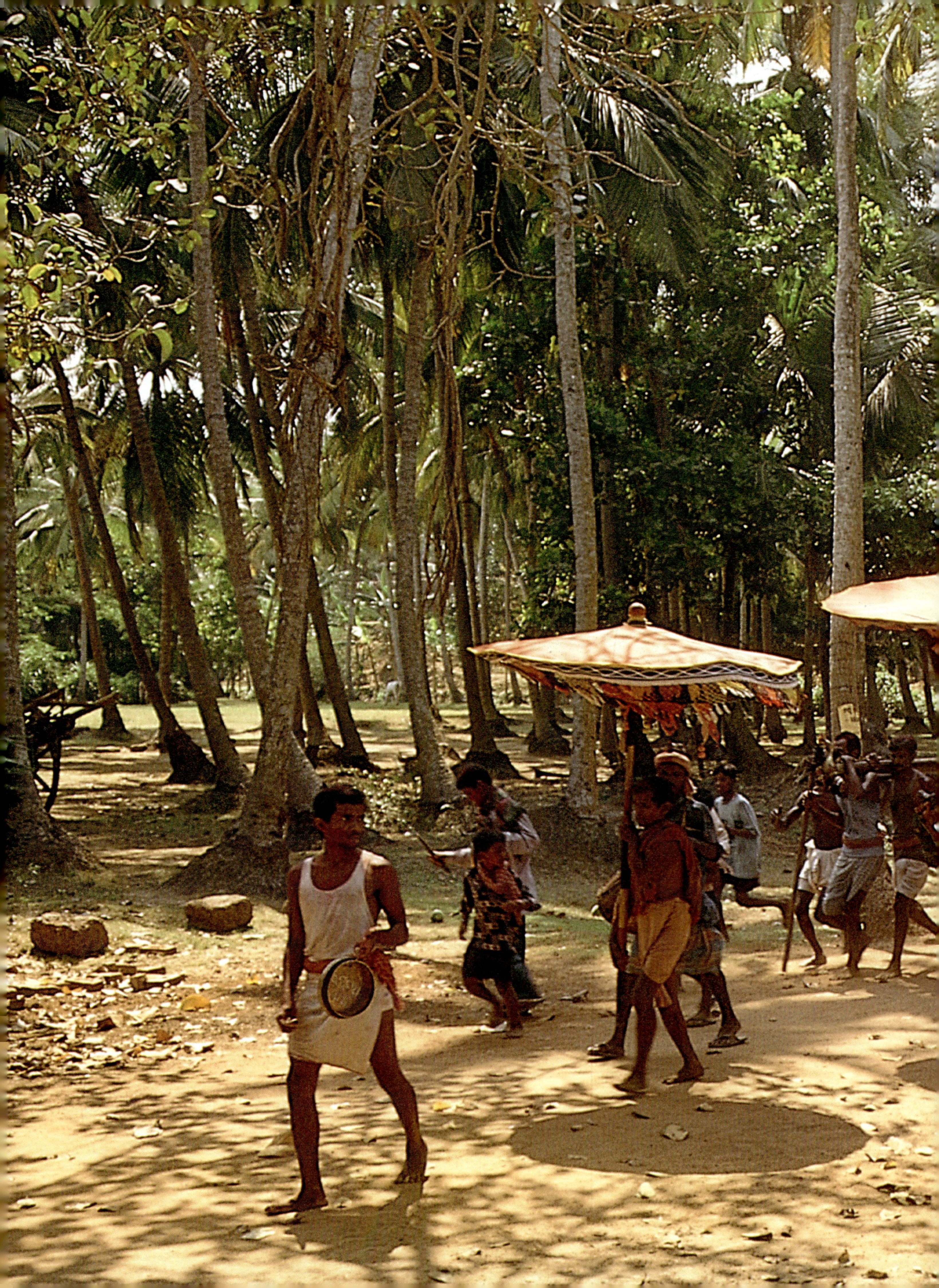

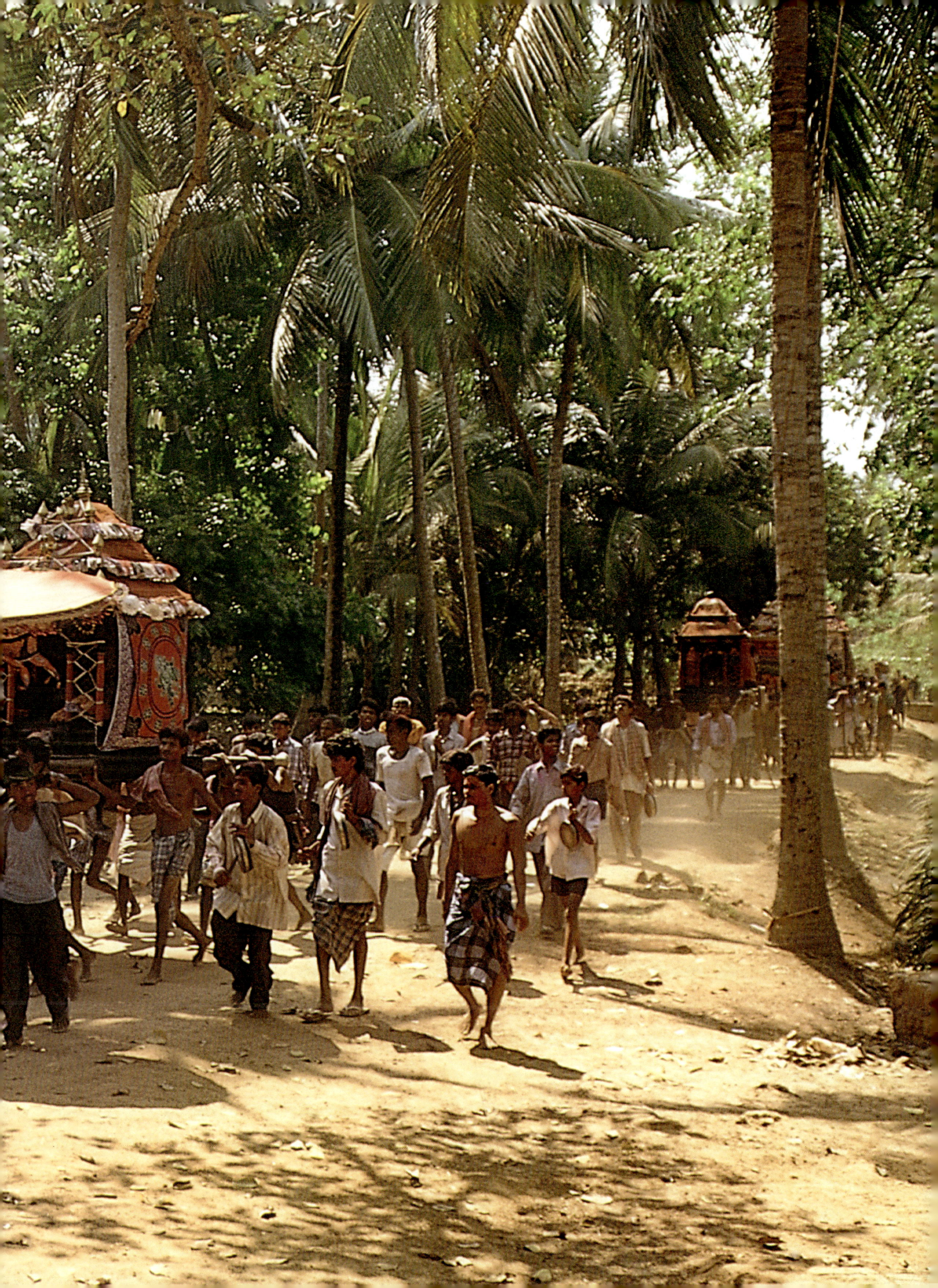

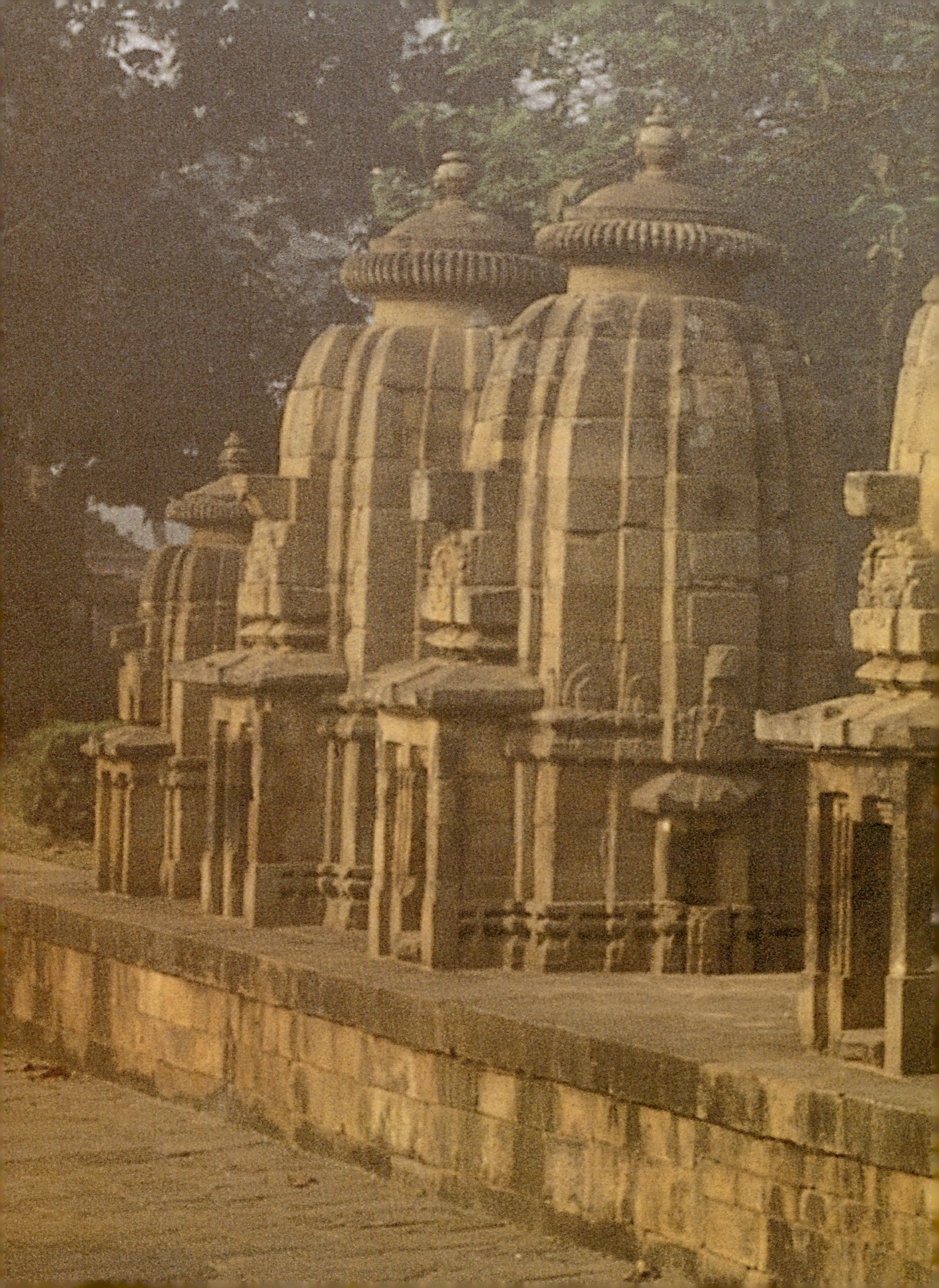

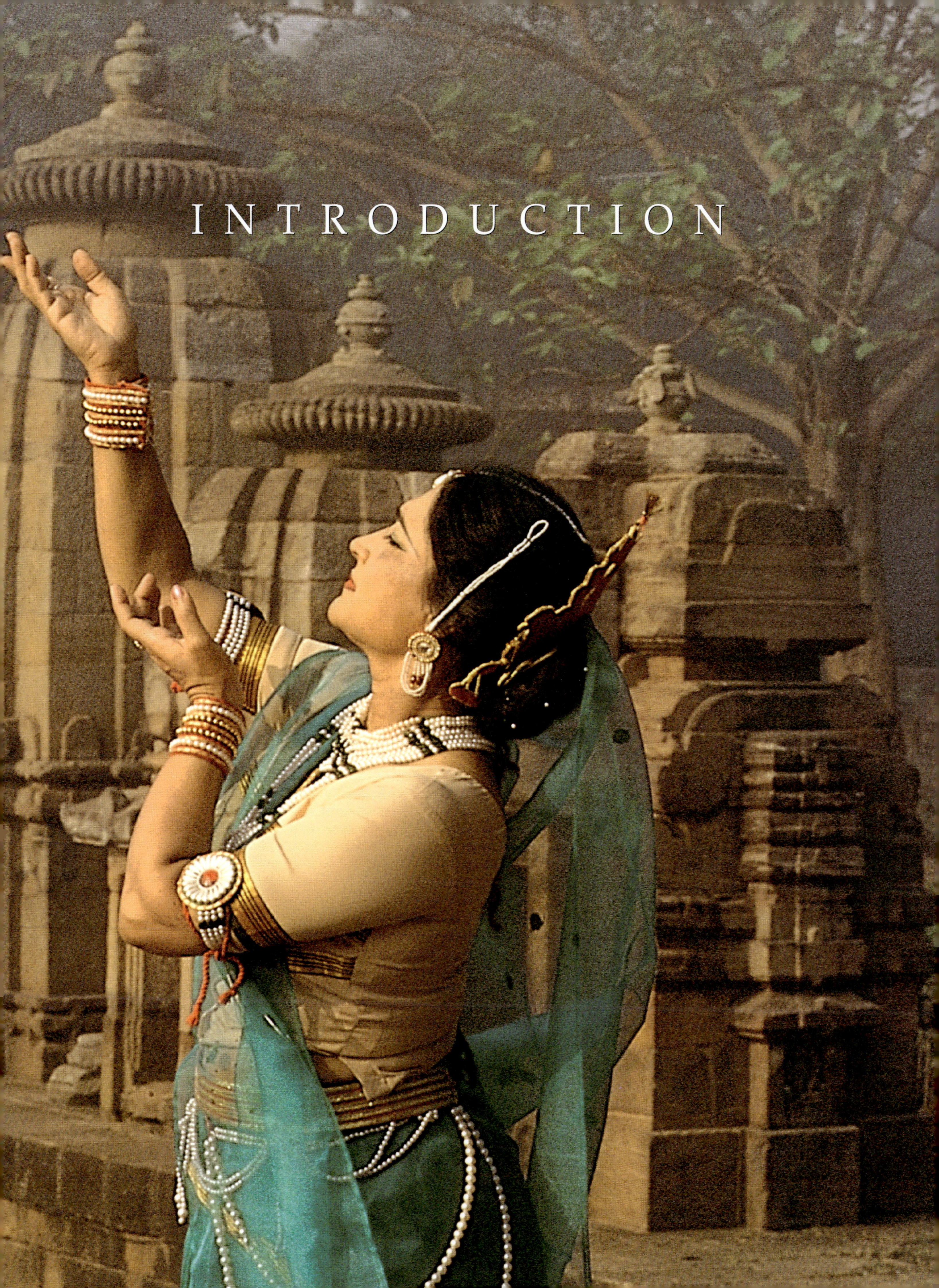

INTRODUCTION

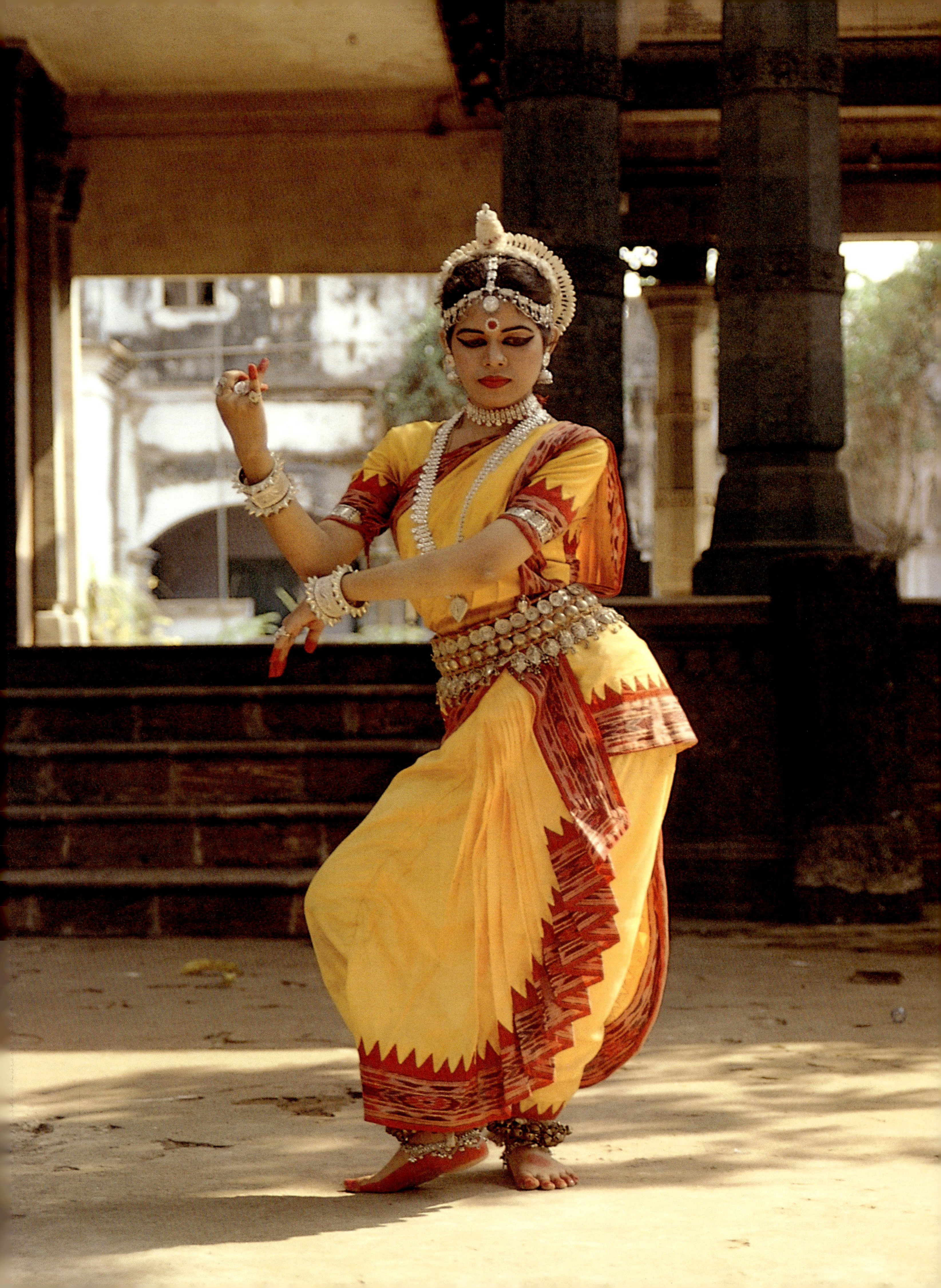

Bharata Muni's *Natya Shastra*, the ancient Sanskrit treatise written about 2000 years ago on the performing arts, describes four regional styles of dance—*avanti, dakshinatya, panchali* and *odhramagadhi*. The *odhramagadhi* style was prevalent in the regions of Odhra, Magadha, Pundra, Kalinga and certain other parts of eastern India. Odhra and Kalinga form the present state of Orissa. It is thus evident that a highly evolved form of classical art was established in this part of India during the ancient times.

चतुर्विधा प्रवृत्तिश्च प्रोक्ता नाट्यप्रयोगतः।।
आवन्ती दाक्षिणात्या च पाञ्चाली चौड्रमागधी।।

Chaturvidha pravrutischa prokta natyaprayogataha II
Aavanti dakshinatya cha panchali chodramagadhi II
—II 13/25, Chapter II, *Natya Shastra*

Taking into consideration the applied aspects of dance, the styles can be divided into four types: *avanti, dakshini, panchali,* and *odhramagadhi*.

The present day Odissi dance evolved out of the *odhramagadhi* performing art form of the yore.

Kaishiki

In *Natya Shastra*, Bharata Muni has described that the *vritti* (character) of *odhramagadhi* is Kaishiki as this is a dance full of *lasya* (feminine, delicate element). All its four *angas* (aspects) are according to the Kaishiki *vritti*.

The Kaishiki *vritti* is described in the *shlokas* (verses) 44-46 (below), Chapter II, *Natya Shastra*:

दीयतां भगवन्द्रव्यं कैशिक्याः सम्प्रयोजकम्।
नृत्ताङ्गहारसम्पन्ना रसभावक्रियात्मिका।।

दृष्टा मया भगवतो नीलकण्ठस्य नृत्यतः।
कैशिकी श्लक्ष्णनैपथ्या श्रृङ्गाररससम्भवा।।

अशक्या पुरुषैः सा तु प्रयोक्तुं स्त्रीजनाहते।
ततोऽसृजन्महातेजा मनसाऽप्सरसो विभुः।।

Left:
A dancer striking a pose in tribhangi.

Following double spread:
A carved wall full of sculptured poses, Sun Temple, Konark.

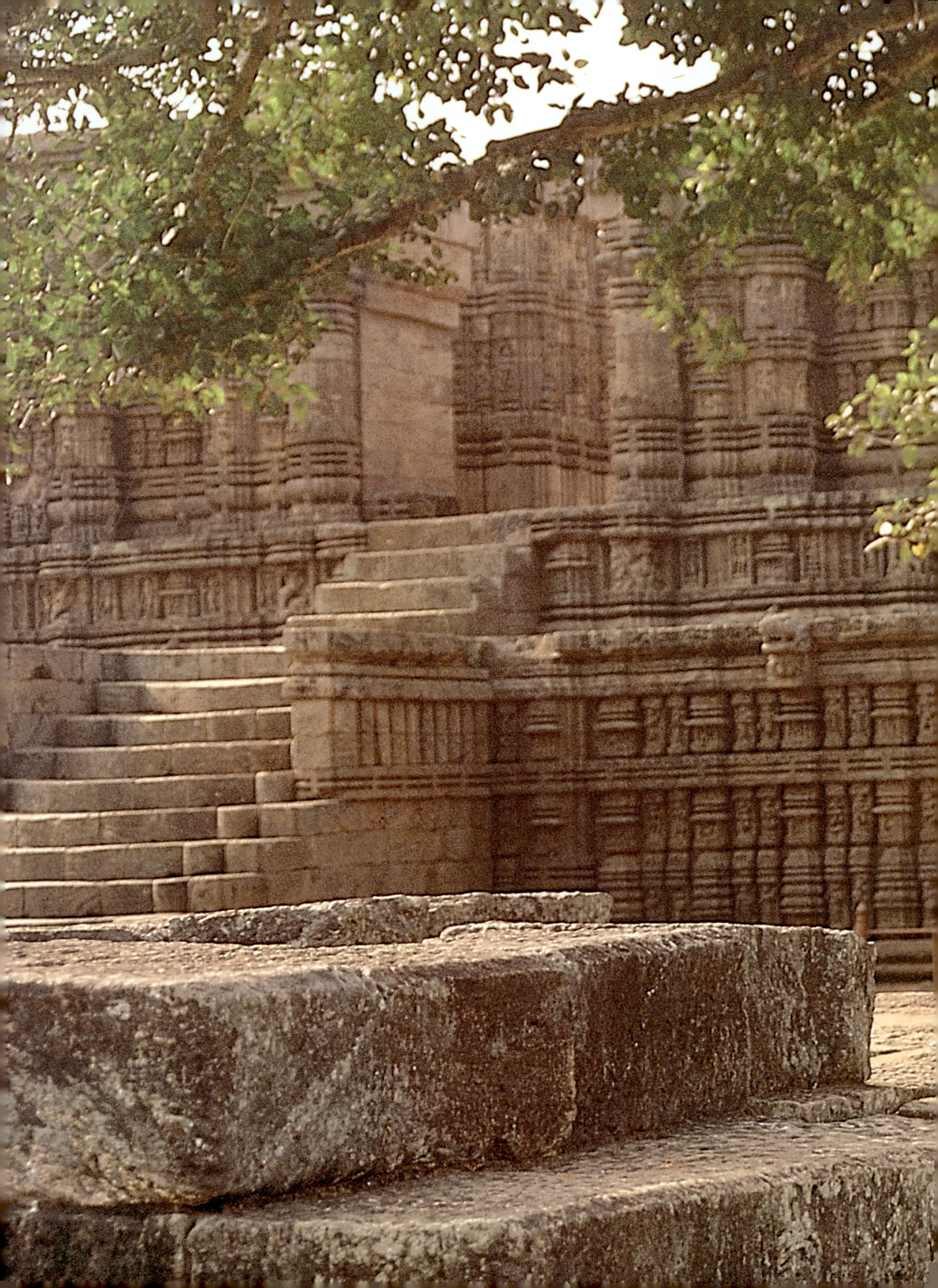

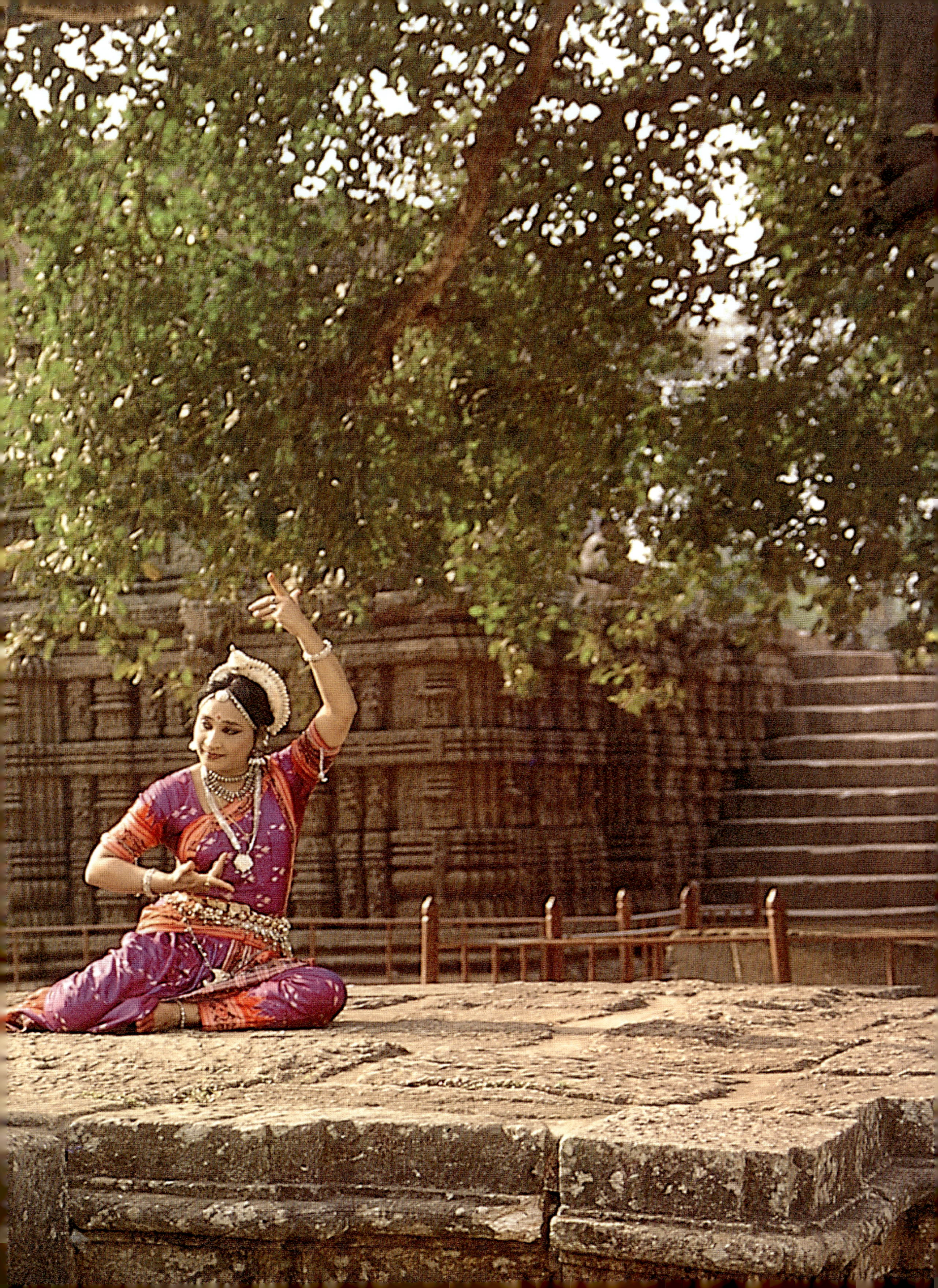

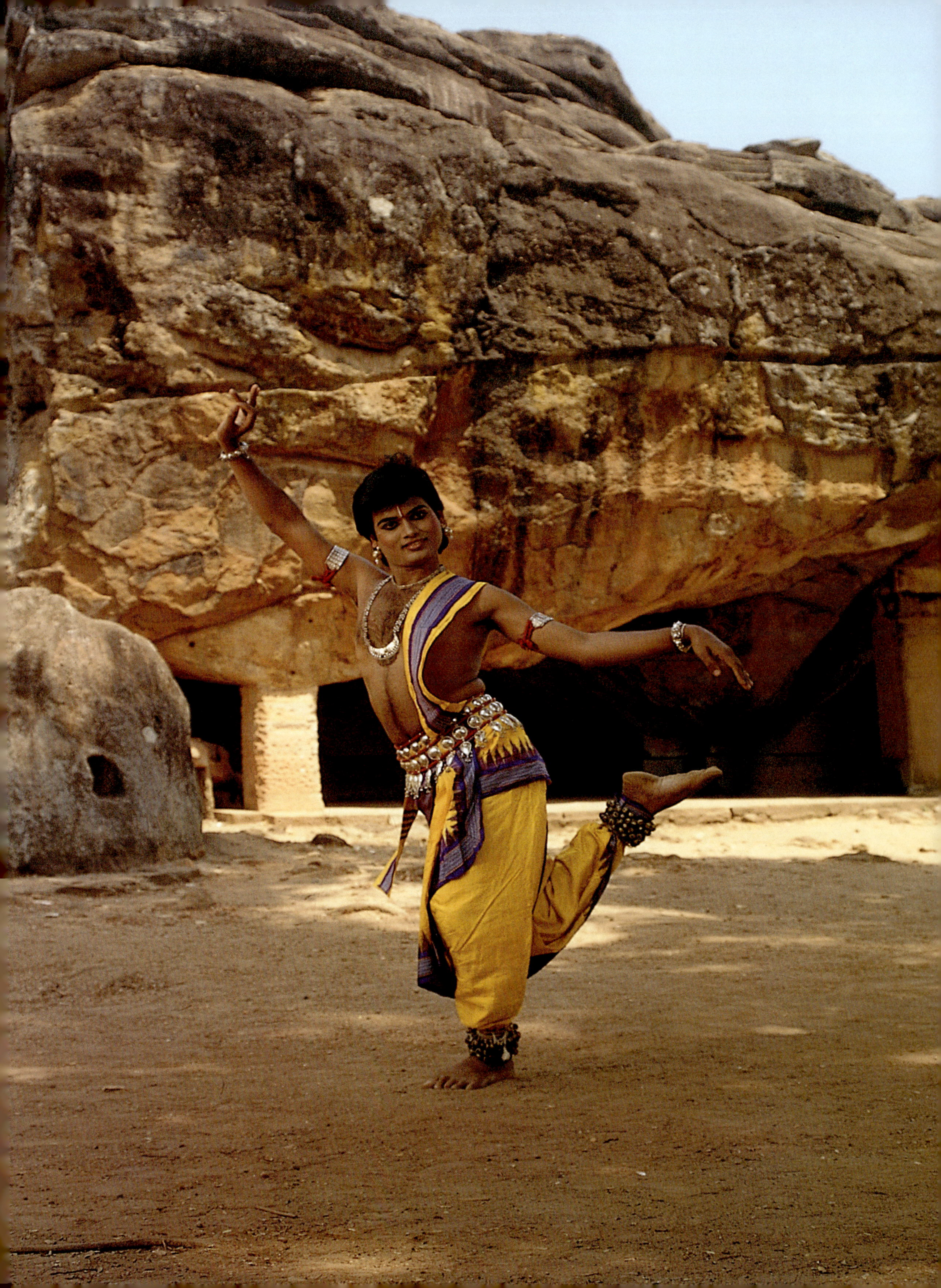

Diyanta bhagavandravyam kaishikyah samprayojakam
Nrityangaharsampanna rasabhavkriyatmika II 44 II

Drushta maya bhagavato nilakanthasya nrutyataha
Kaishiki shralakshanepathya shrungararasambhava II 45 II

Ashakya purushyah sa tu prayokantum strijanahate
Tatohsrujanmahateja mansahpasarso vibhuha II 46 II

Kaishiki has power to create *sringara rasa.* This *vritti* is one where the artistes are mostly women, wearing charming and colourful costumes; where there is plenty of dancing and music, and the theme is of love and its enjoyment. Conclusively, Odissi conforms to the graceful style of Kaishiki dance as described in the *Natya Shastra*.

Rich in substance and intensity of emotions, Odissi is a beautiful and rare synthesis of sensuousness and devotion. Sculptures in the temples of Orissa come alive in the movements as the rhythm of dance is captured in thousands of images adorning these temples. This sculpturesque quality is perhaps the most striking feature of Odissi.

Left: A young male dancer depicting Krishna and his chakra.

Below: A mahari *dancer.*

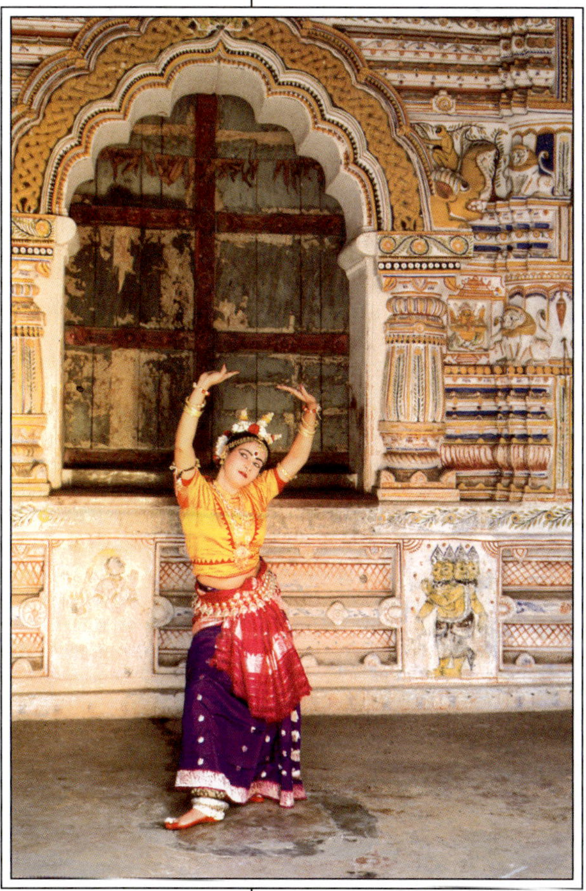

The dance form grew from the tradition of the *mahari*, or the temple dancer, who served the Lord in the Jagannath Temple. The influence of Jagannath, the Lord of the Universe (synonymous with Krishna), is so pronounced that Odissi stands apart from other classical dance forms owing to its devotional expression and predominance of the Krishna theme.

Odissi is arguably the most lyrical style of Indian classical dance. Charles Fabri, the Hungarian Indologist credited with being one of the first to rediscover Odissi, considered it to be 'the most perfect Indian classical dance form'.

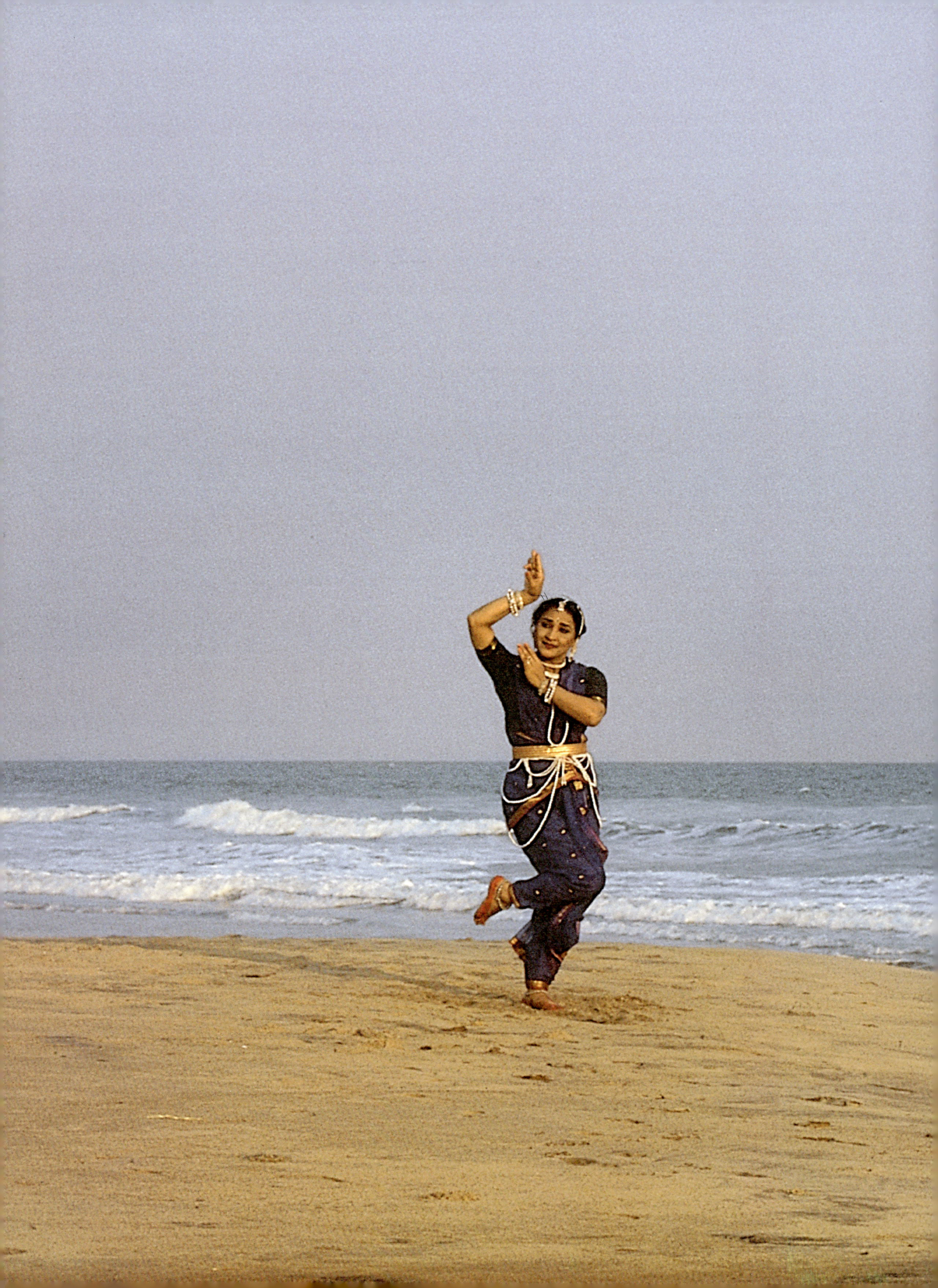

THE BIRTH OF DANCE

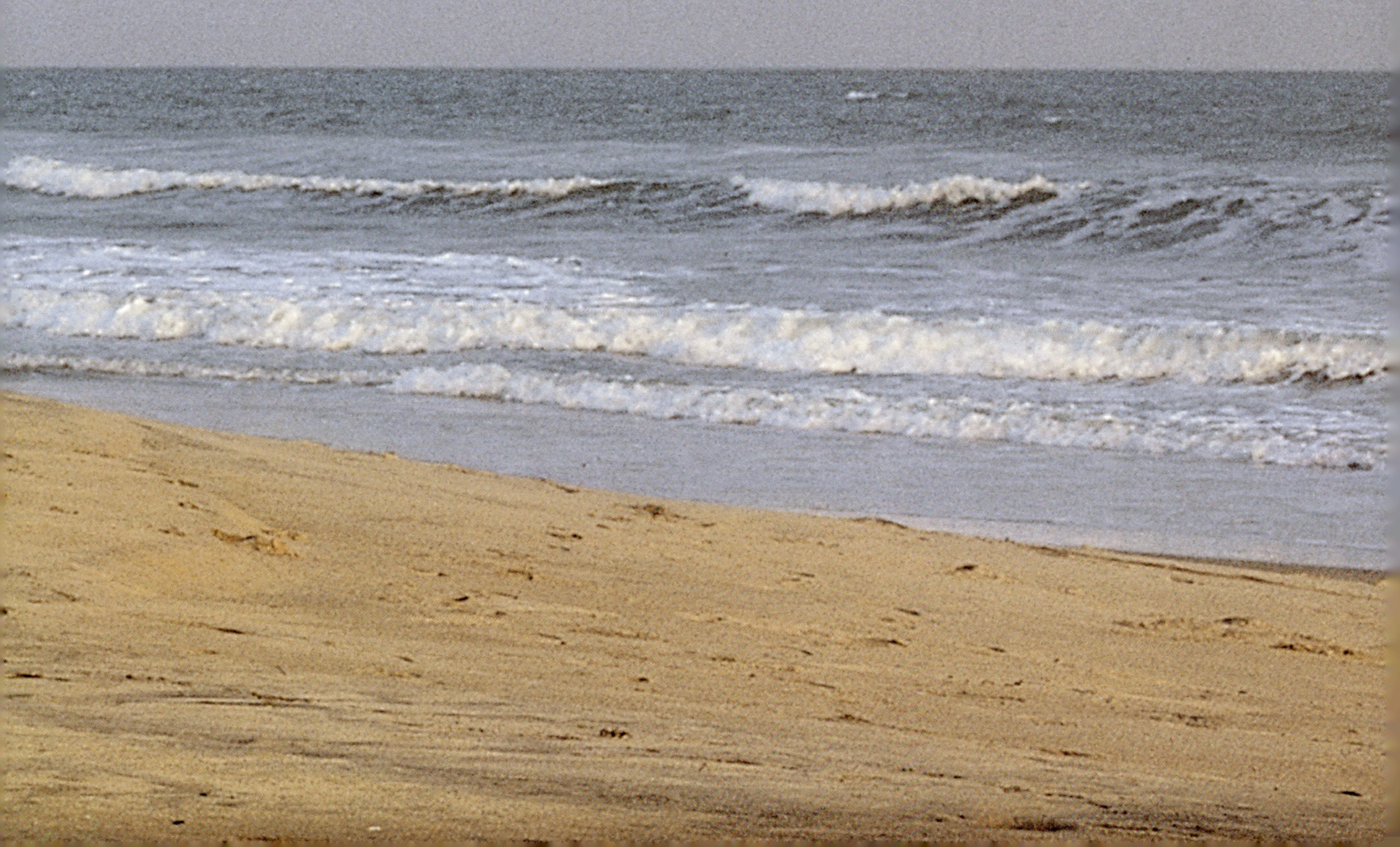

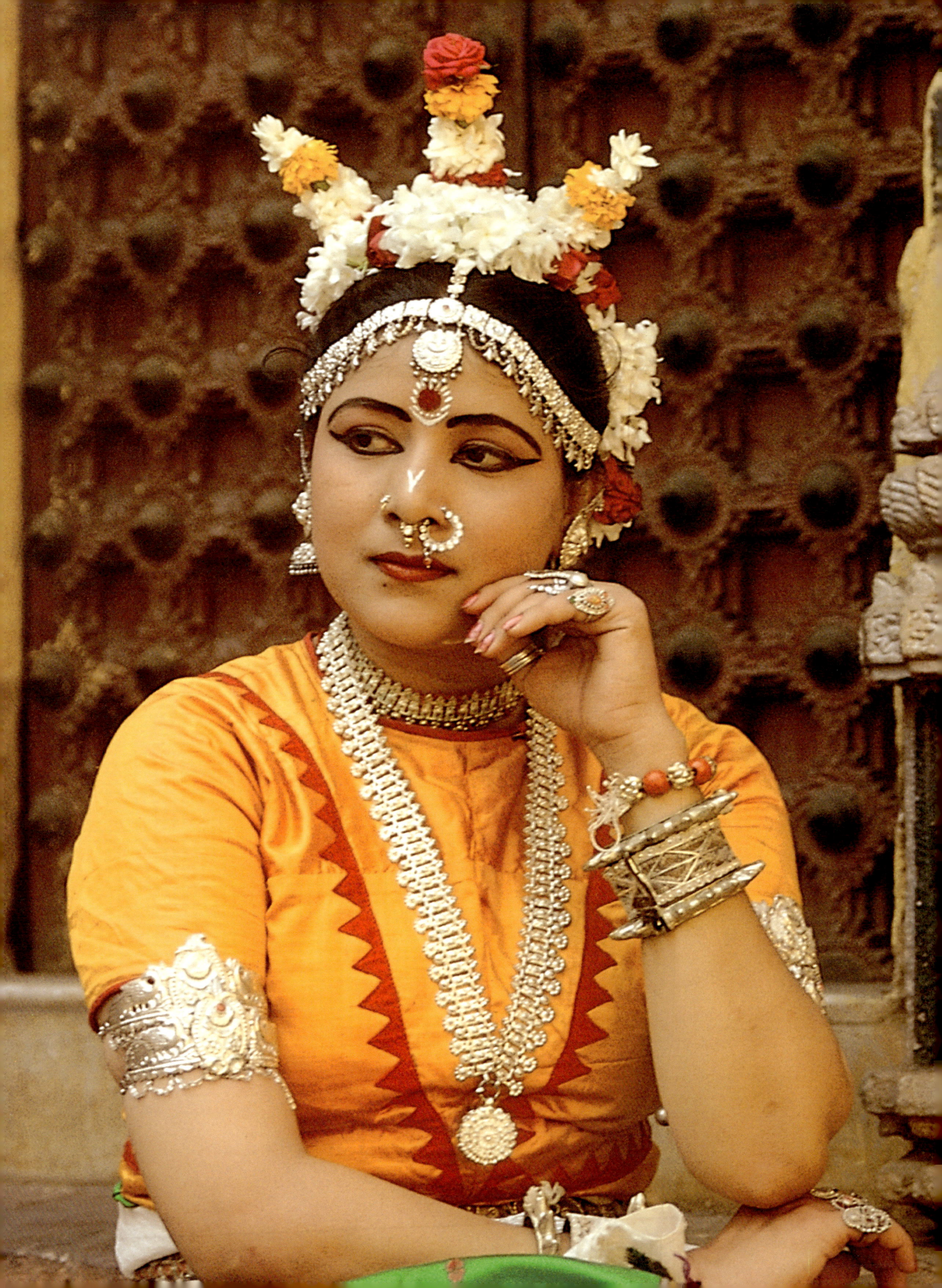

Long long ago, when the gods and the demons wanted to obtain *amrit* or ambrosia which would ensure immortality, they churned the *samudra*—the ocean— in tandem to beget it.

They decided to use the mountain, Mandara, as the churning rod which they placed on the back of Akupara, the Divine Turtle. To churn the great mountain they used the Divine Serpent, Vasuki, as the rope.

The gods held the serpent from one side and the demons on the other. They churned the ocean first one way, then the other. The waters began to twist, slowly at first, but then faster, till they began to surge in huge waves.

From the *samudra manthan*, came *amrit* and along with *amrit* came many other wonderous things. Most wonderous among them were beautiful *apsaras.*

They were blessed with youthfulness and grace.

They were adept in dancing and singing.

They inspired love in paradise as well as on earth.

They had the ability to divert men from their ascetic practices.

They adored Kamadeva, the God of Love.

They moved to heaven and became dancers in Indra's court.

Gandharvas, renowned musicians, bards and singers, were consorts to these celestial nymphs.... .

When they played on their divine instruments, the *apsaras,* danced.... .

And thus began the tradition of dance according to Indian mythology.

It is said that once when an *apsara* known as Urvasi was performing an enchanting dance before Indra, her eyes met the impassioned gaze of Jayanta, the son of Indra, and for a moment, her mind was diverted from her dance.

On seeing this, the sage Agastya, became angry and cursed them both.

Urvasi was to be born on earth as a *devadasi*—temple dancer—and Jayanta as a bamboo tree on the Vindya Hills.

Urvasi and Jayanta fell at the feet of the great sage and begged him to retract his curse. Agastya relented and made the curse less harsh. He decried that when Urvasi would perform her debut dance in the temple before the gods, she would be presented with a staff fashioned from the bamboo tree of Jayanta in the Vindya Hills. When this happened, the curse would be lifted and Urvasi and Jayanta would ascend to heaven. Urvasi took birth on the earth as a *devadasi* and taught the art of dance to beautiful women.

Thus started the tradition of the *devadasi* dancing on earth.... .

Left: Portrait of a contemporary mahari *dancer.*

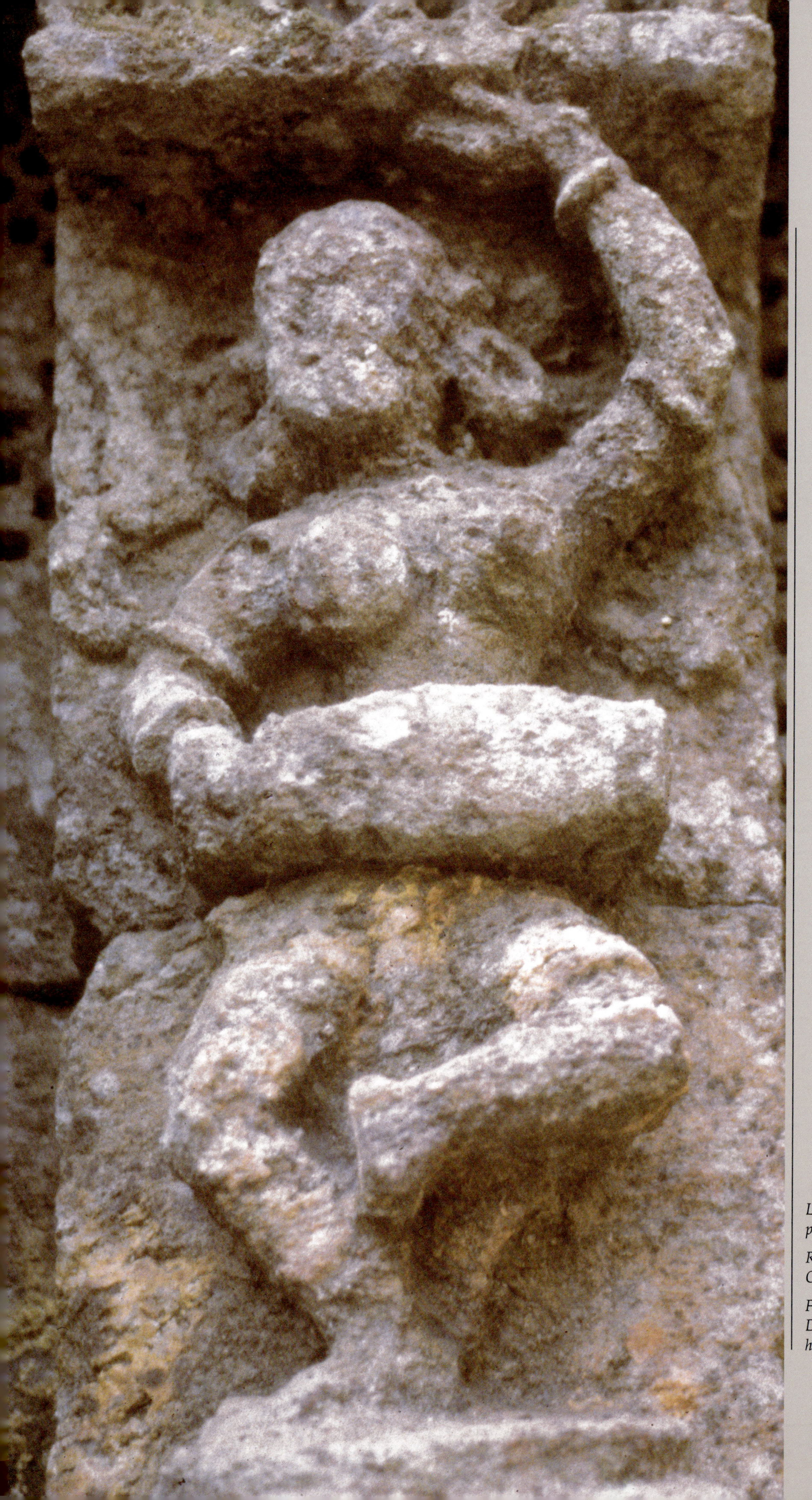

Left: Sculpture of a mardala *player, Konark Temple.*

Right: Depicting alasya, *an Odissi dance posture.*

Following double spread: Depicting lovebirds by hand gesture.

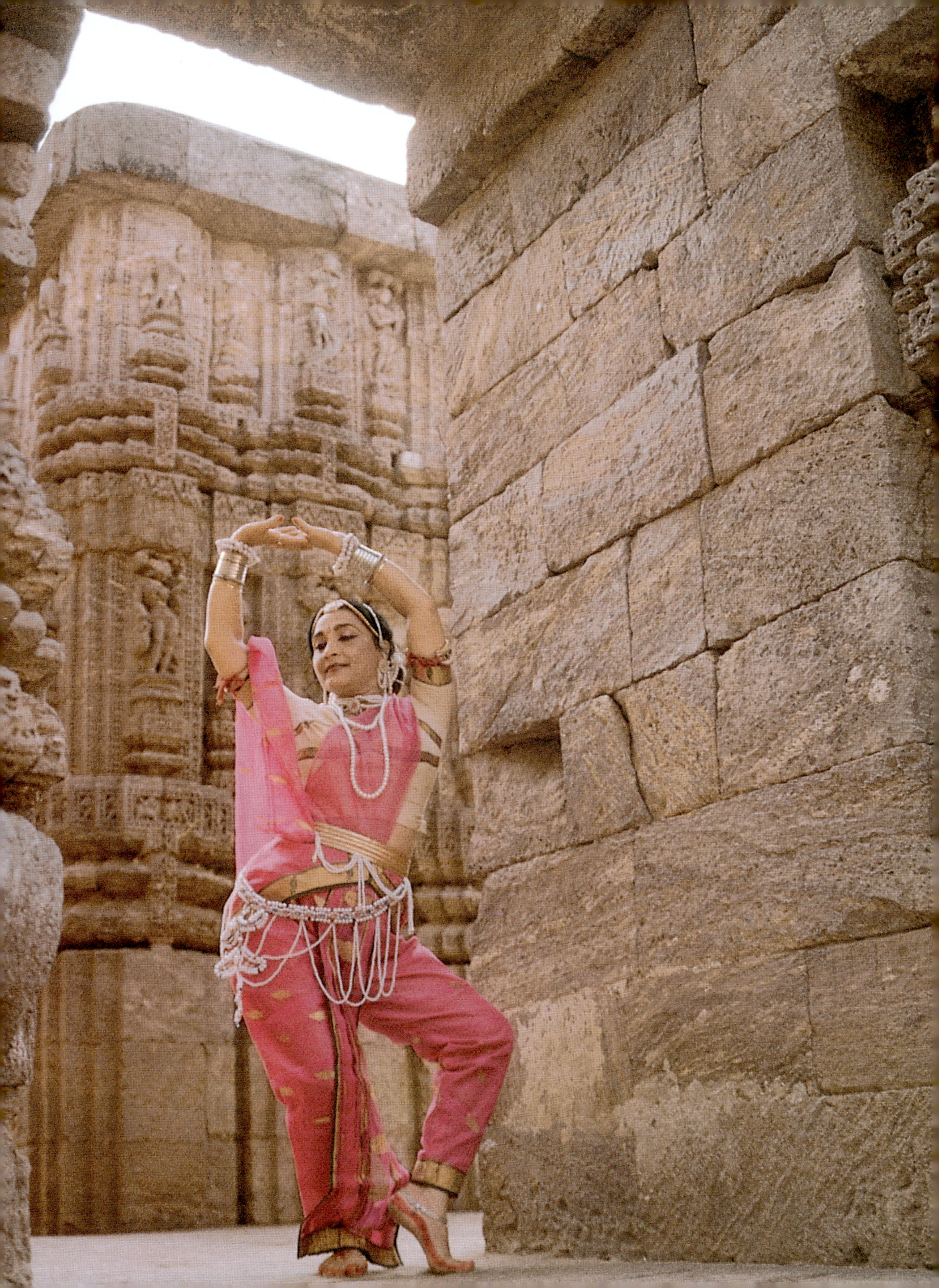

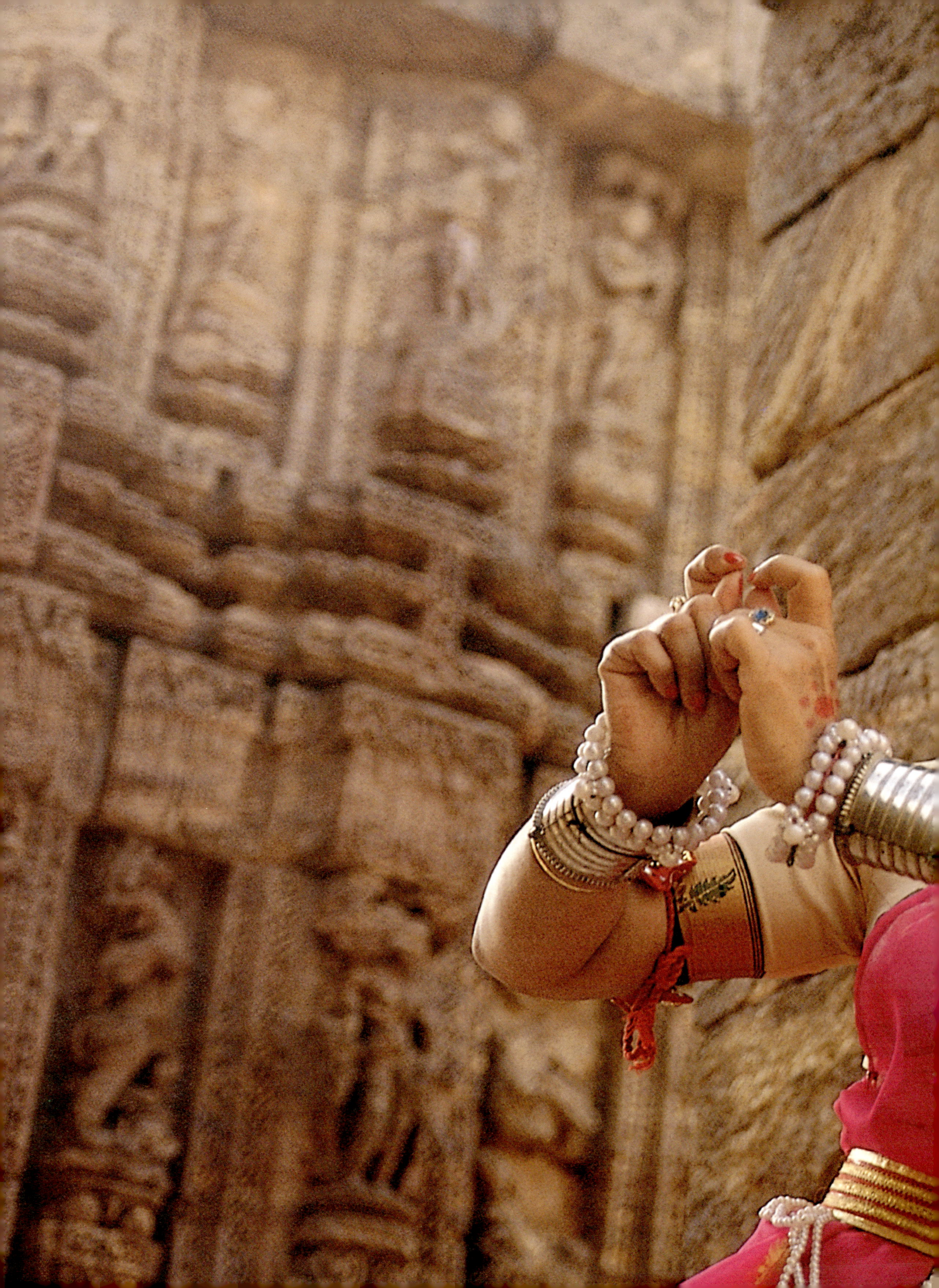

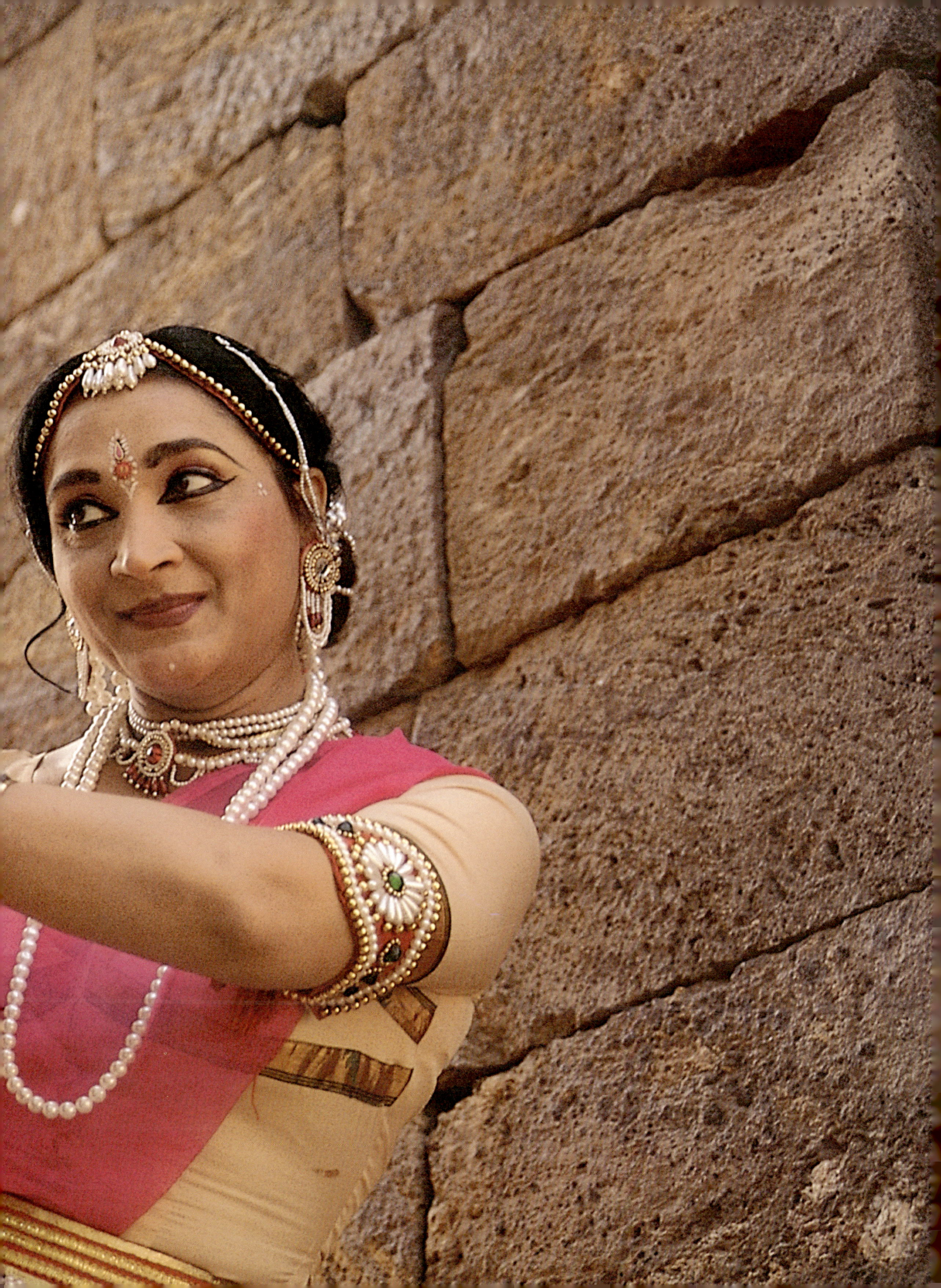

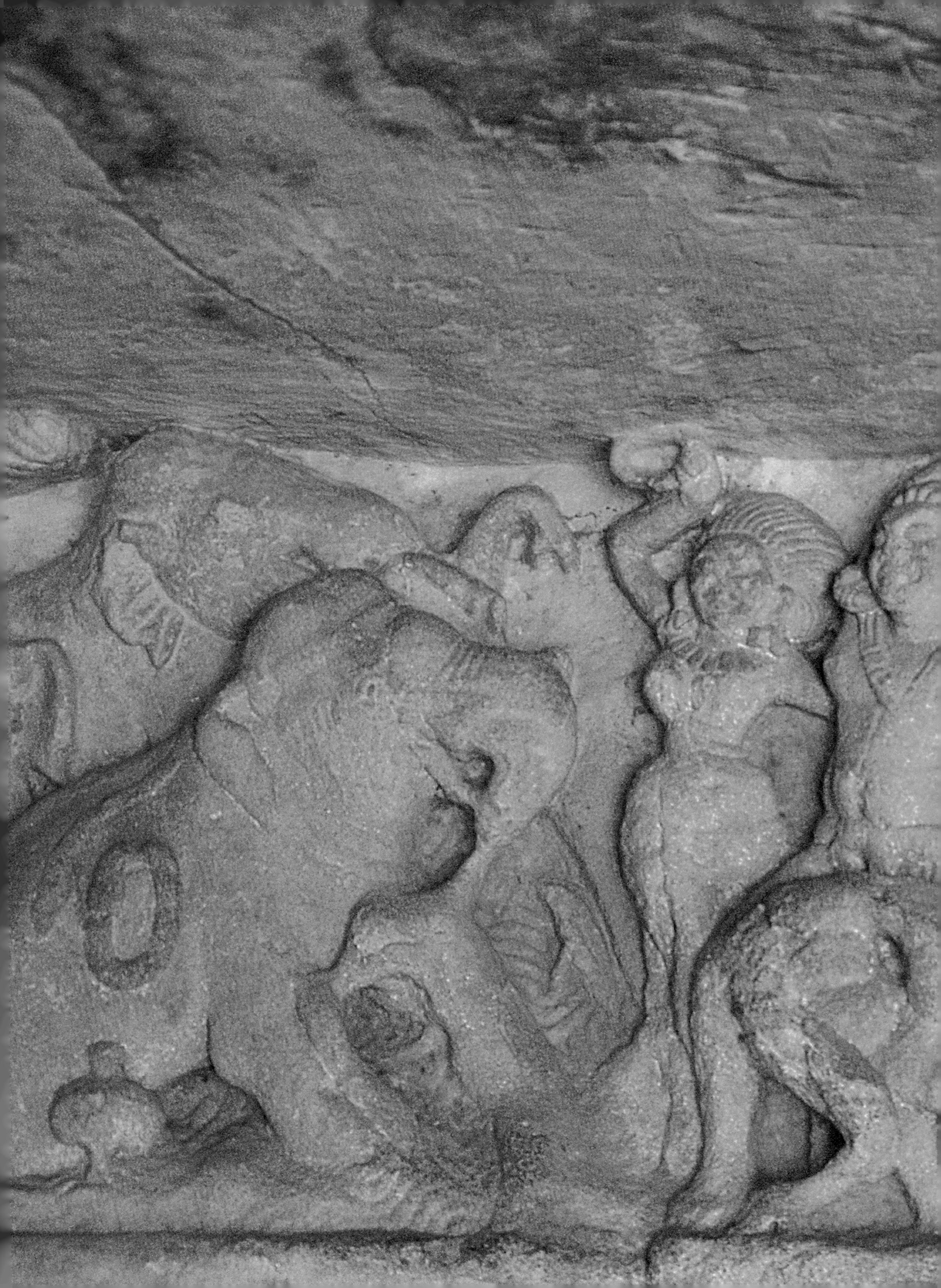

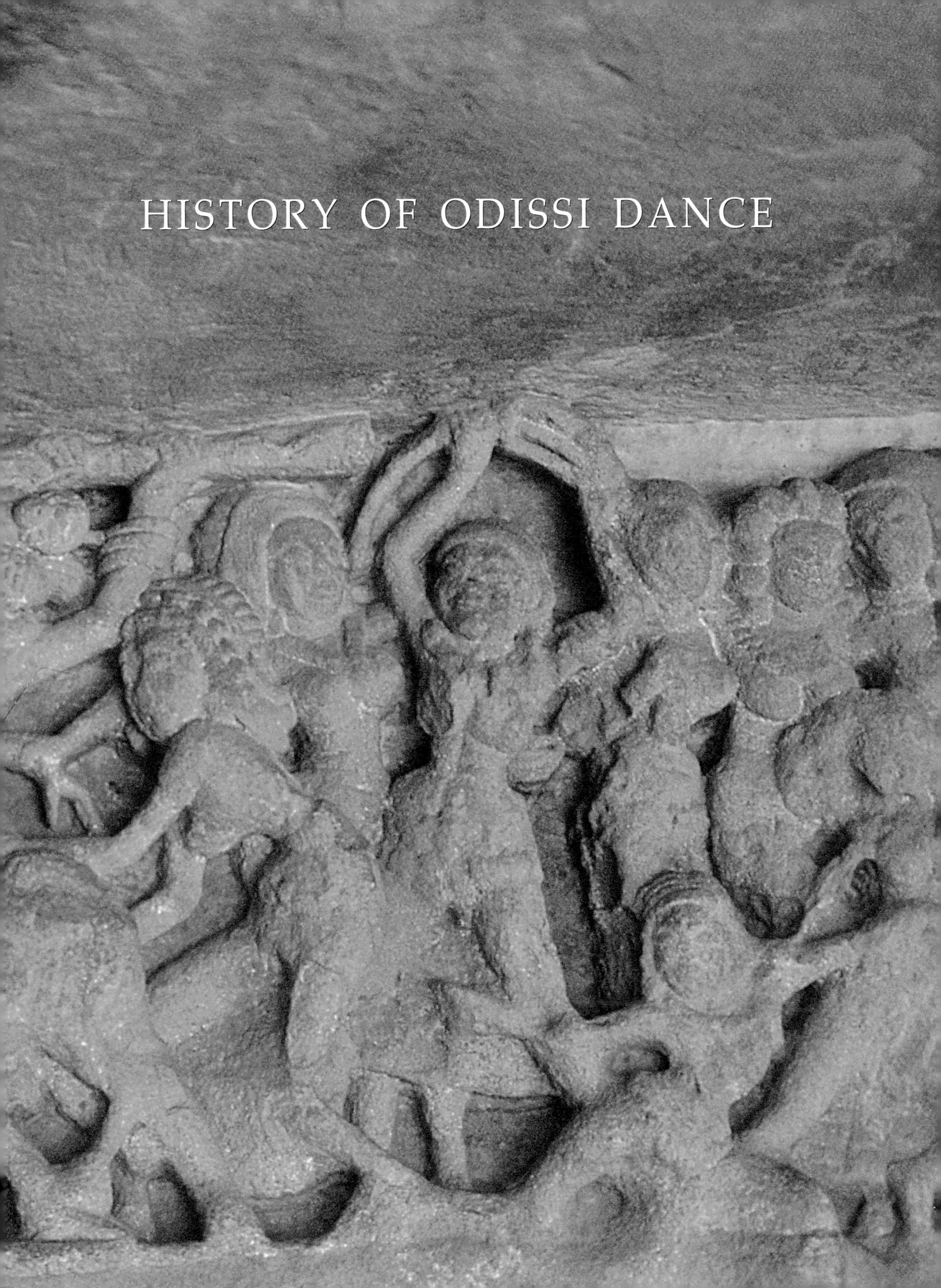
HISTORY OF ODISSI DANCE

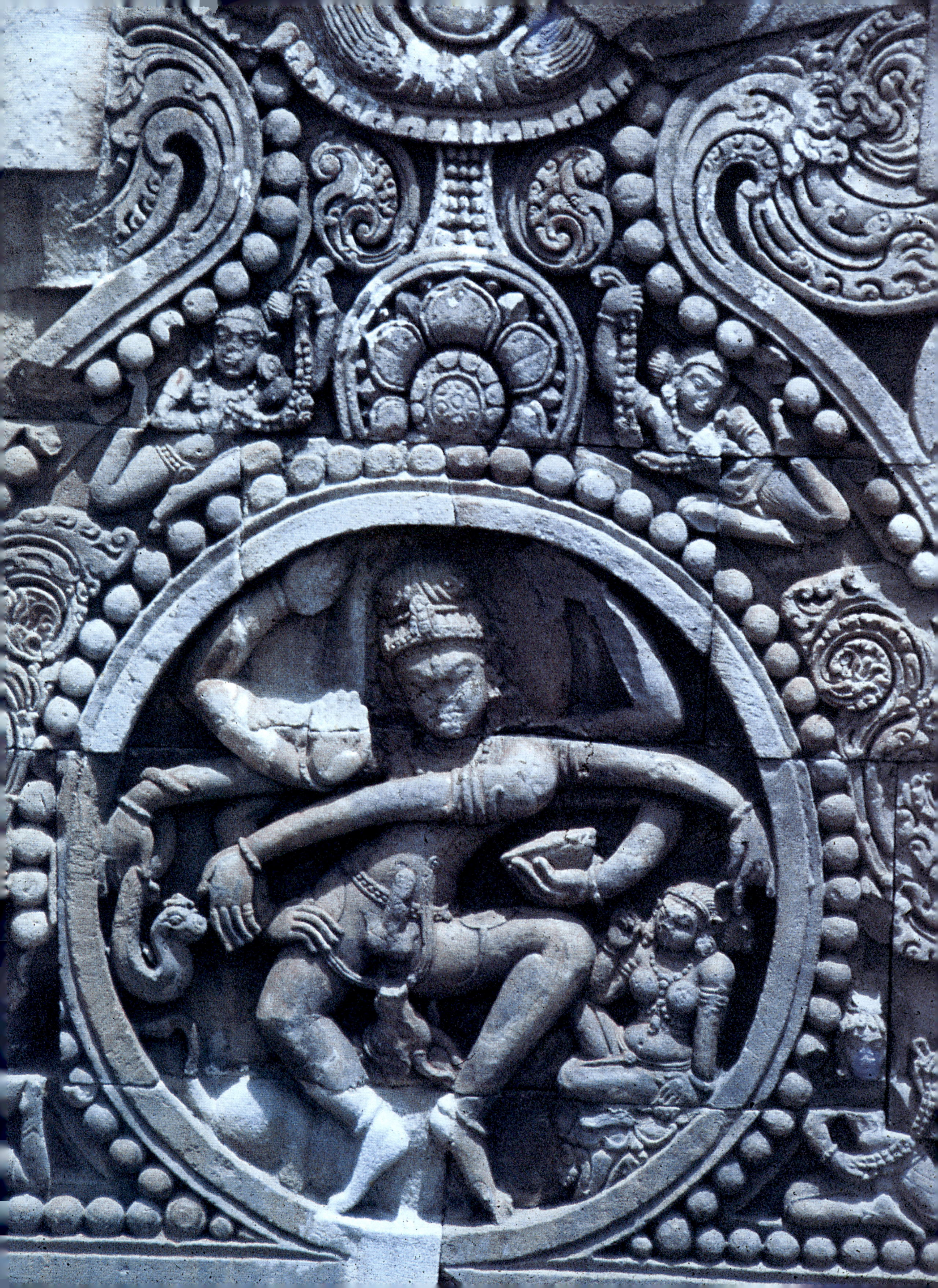

Though the origin of Indian classical dance is widely understood and accepted in mythological terms, the first historical and archaeological evidence of Odissi dance was found in the cave sculptures of the Udayagiri and Khandagiri hills near Bhubaneswar in Orissa. Built around the 1st century BC by the Jain king Kharavela, the caves are engraved with inscriptions and sculptures that prove the significance of the arts in the lives of the people of Kalinga, the ancient name of Orissa.

King Kharavela is known and remembered for being an extremely wealthy and successful ruler, a devout Jain, and a great patron of the arts. The *Ranigumpha*—the Queen's Cave—is adorned with a multitude of panels and sculptures that celebrate the artistic lifestyle of King Kharavela's times. Numerous musicians and beautiful dancers in different poses are found in these images, the most famous of which is the sculpture of the dancer known as the *nartaki*. The *nartaki*, in its vigorous and proud stance, bears a remarkable resemblance to a posture from the contemporary dance form. For the Odissi dancers of today, the *nartaki* has become a landmark of the ancient-in-contemporary continuum of Odissi. It marks the historical evolution of one of the world's most beautiful dance traditions—Odissi.

Preceding double spread: A panel from the Udayagiri Khandagiri Caves depicting a dance performance in the court of King Kharavela.

Left: Shiva as Nataraja, *Parashurameshwara Temple, Bhubaneswar.*

Below: A panel from the Udayagiri Khandagiri Caves.

Following double spread: Sculptures of dancers and stylised animal forms from the Konark Temple.

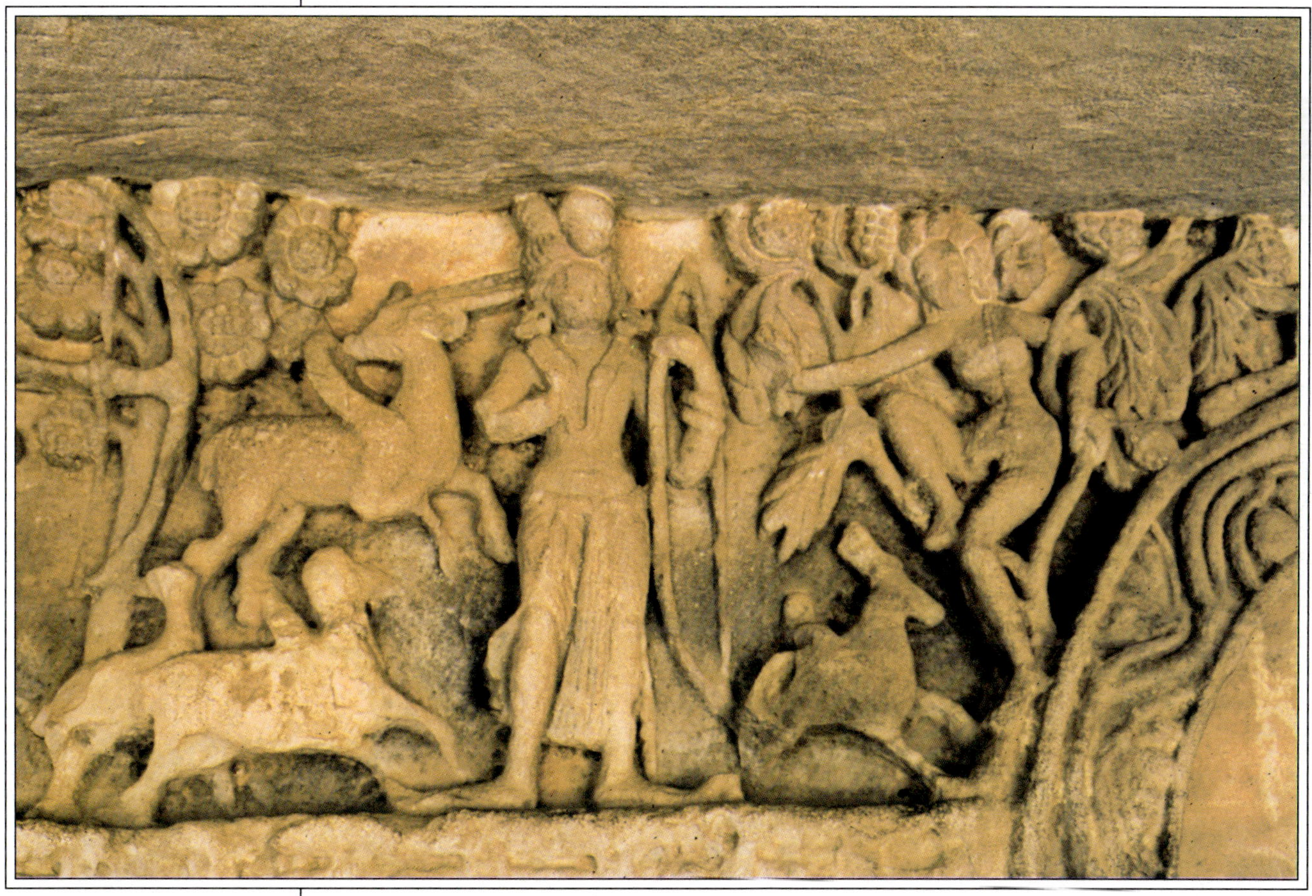

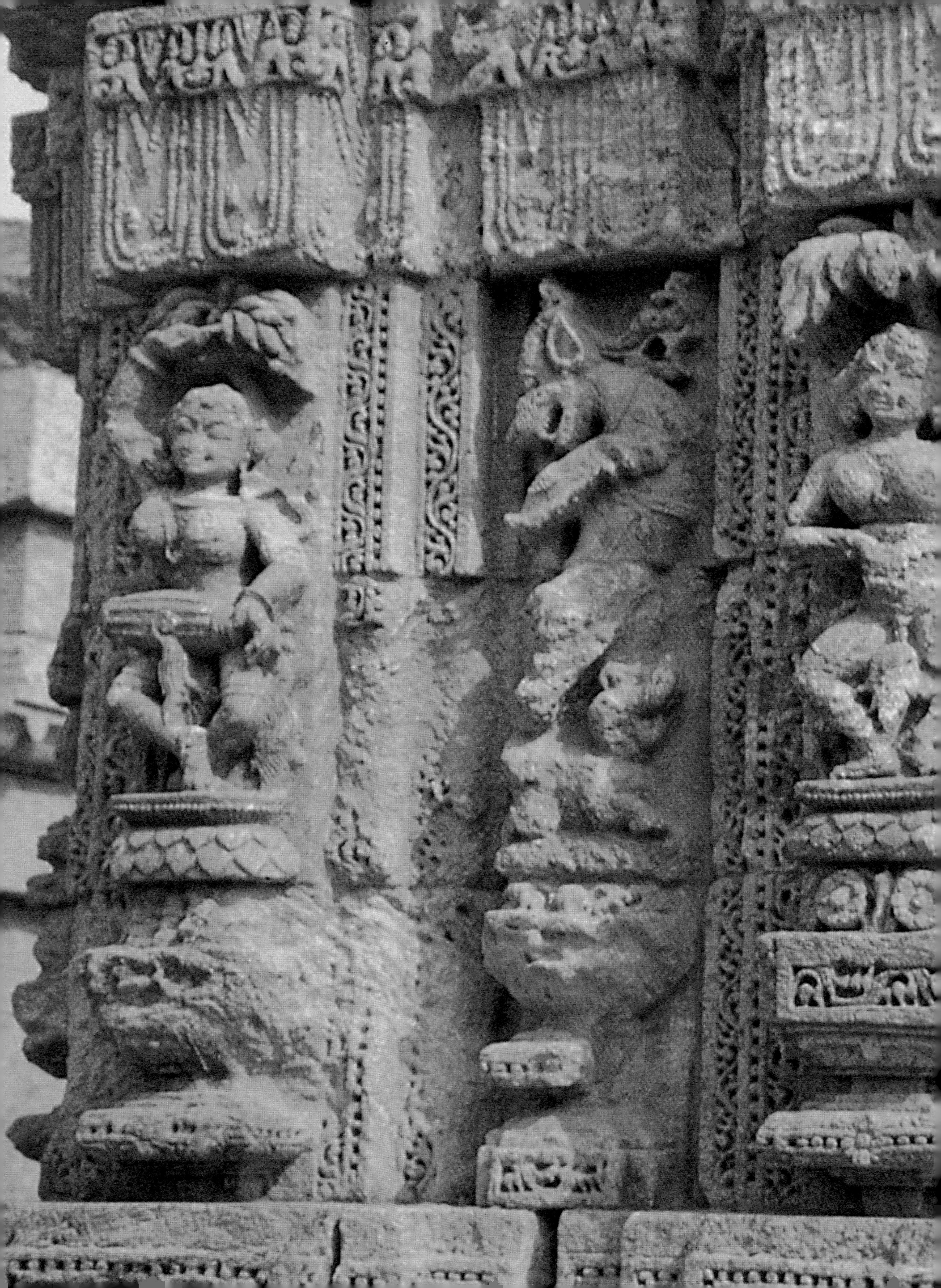

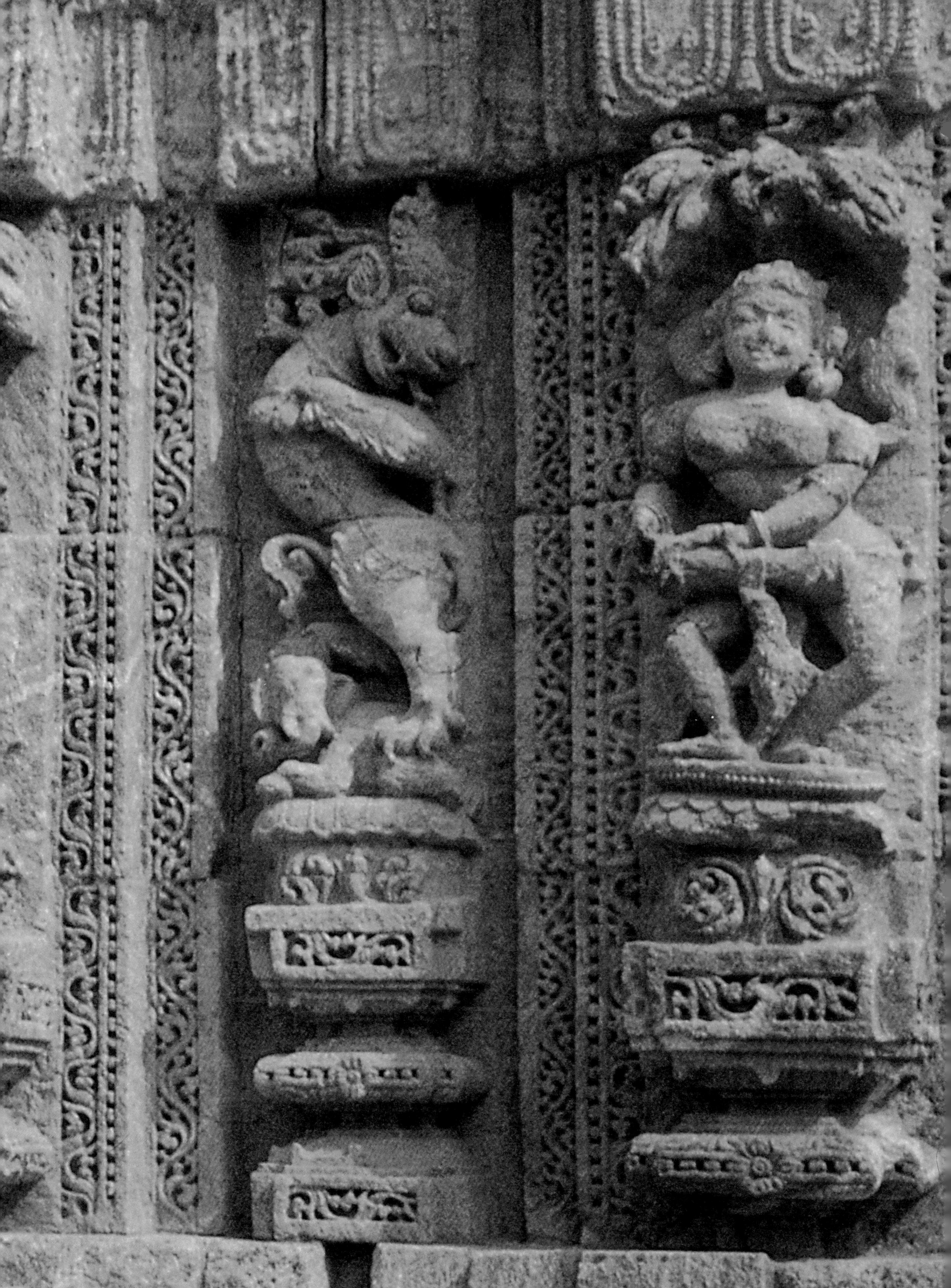

After King Kharavela's death, no clear picture of Oriya history emerges. Although little is known about the history of dance until approximately the 7th century AD, there is evidence to indicate that Kalinga did indeed remain a vibrant and important cultural, artistic and religious centre.

Buddhism, which flourished initially under the 'golden' rule of Ashoka before the time of Kharavela, reasserted itself in Kalinga in the 3rd century AD in its Mahayana form. Mahayana Buddhism is believed to have been aesthetically a very sensitive religion that regarded artistic expression as not merely 'a profession, but a path towards truth and self-realisation, both for the maker and the spectator'. The art of dance, far from forbidden, was celebrated as a means of deliverance and an act of spiritual awareness.

After the fall of the Buddhist kingdoms, the advent of Shaivism forced the followers of Mahayana Buddhism to strive for royal patronage. Though it is unclear how and when Shaivism first entered Orissa, but by the 4th century AD there was evidence to prove the existence of the faith and the religious significance of dance to Shaivites.

A clearer picture of Shaivite history emerges with the rise of the Sailodbhava dynasty in the 7th century. The Sailodbhava kings united a large

Below: A dancer making a flower offering in the courtyard of the Mukteshwar Temple.

Right: Nataraja *with twelve arms at the Mukteshwar Temple.*

Following double spread: Sun Temple, Konark.

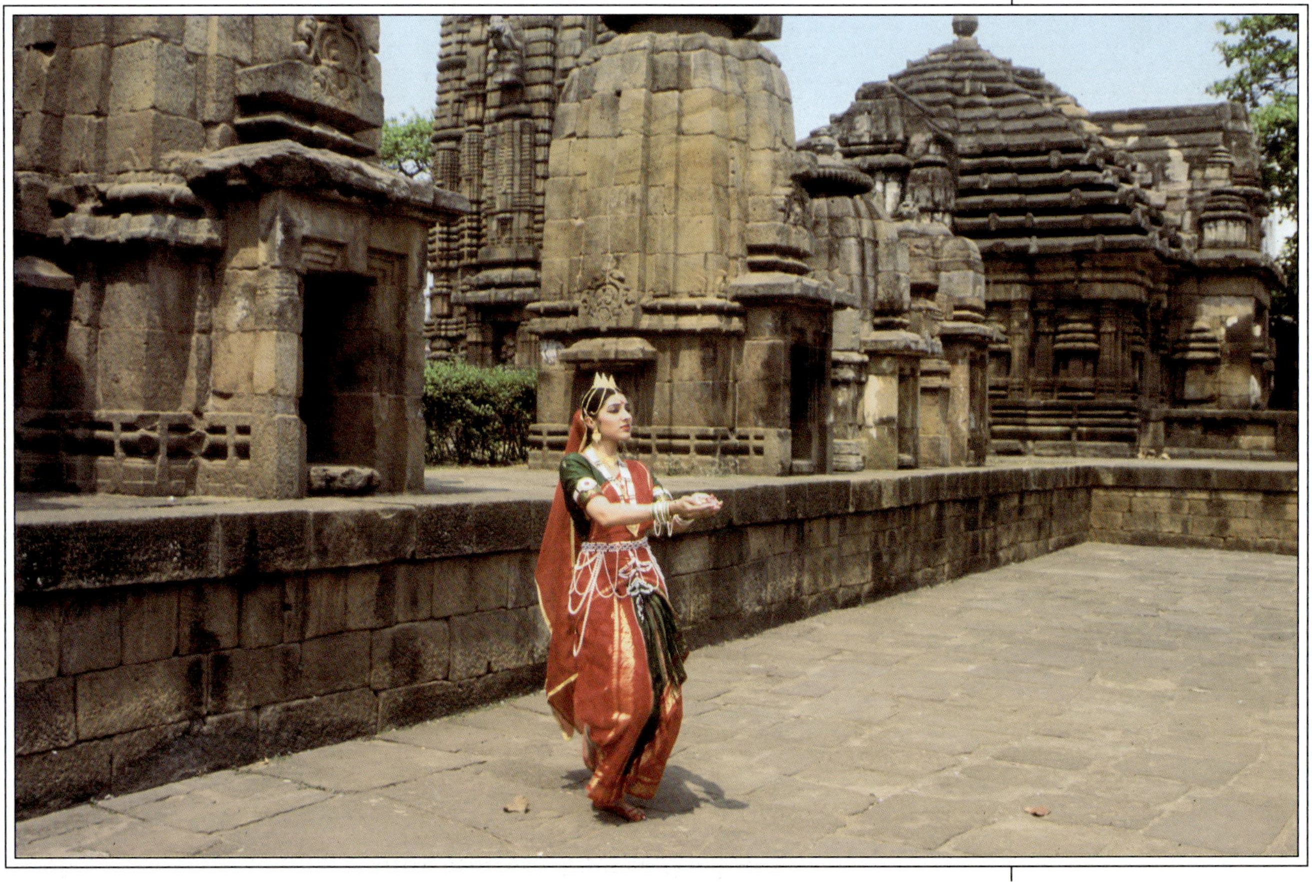

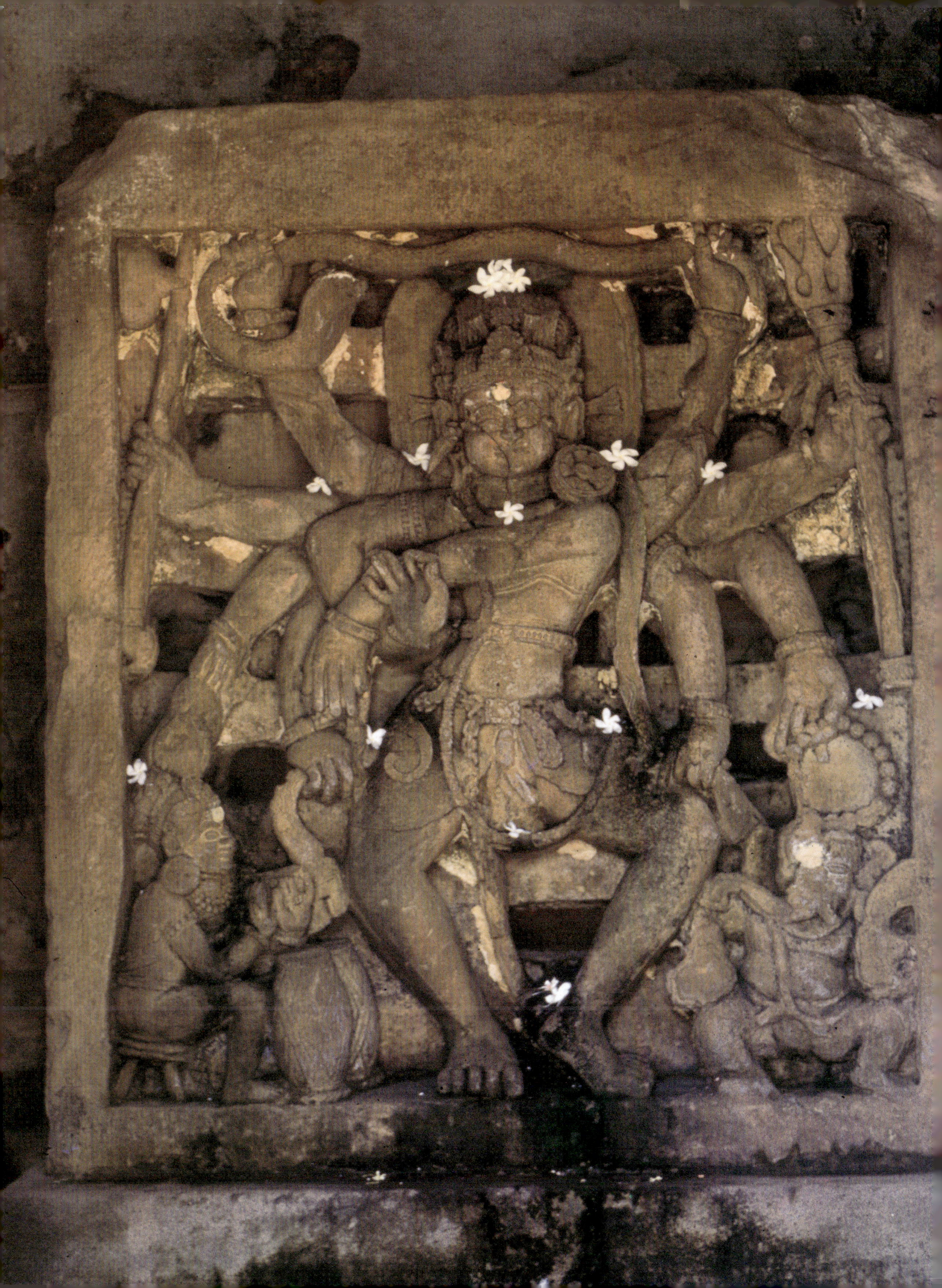

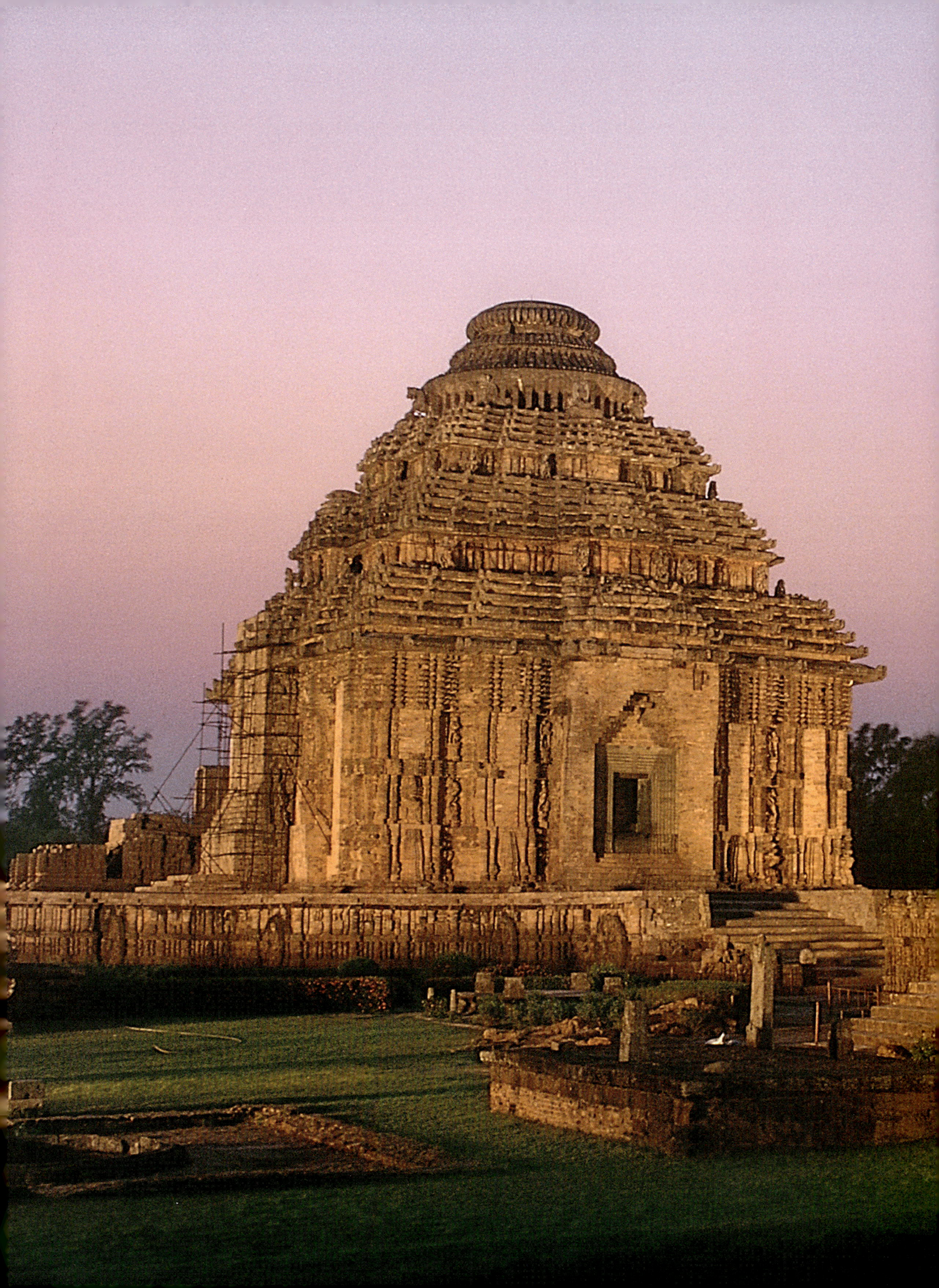

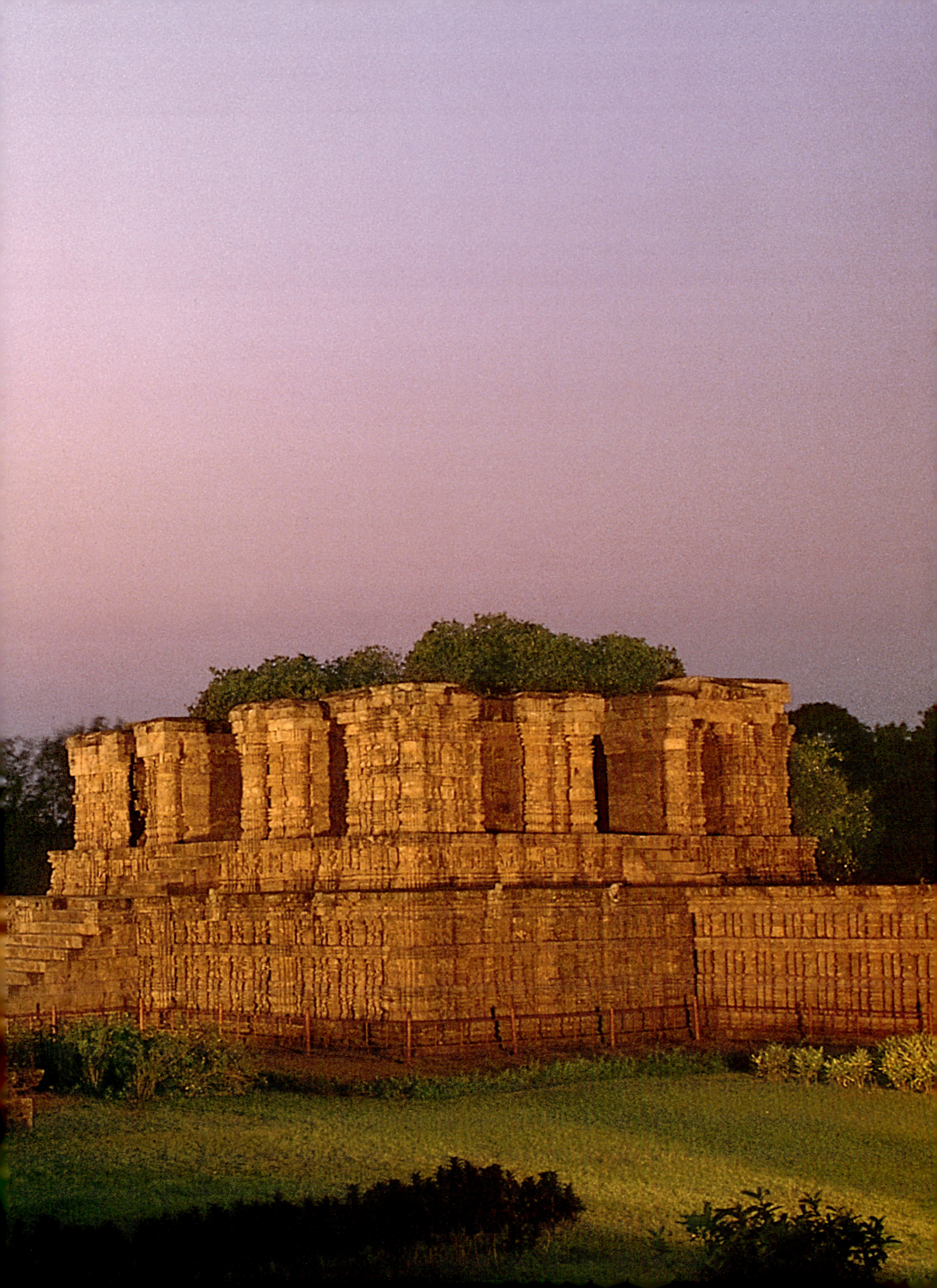

part of ancient Orissa. The era was characterised by a sound system of administration, a sincere tolerance of all religions, a rich tradition of art and culture, and the construction of innumerable temples dedicated to Lord Shiva. Sculptures of dancing girls and images of the dancing Shiva, called *Nataraja*, can be seen in the earliest of the surviving temples of this period, including the Mukteshwar, Parashurameshwara and other temples. These sculptures and the magnificent temples on which they are carved, corroborate the glorification of Shaivism. Fostering a tradition of artistic excellence in architecture, sculpture and dance that was inspired by the Cosmic Dancer himself, Shaivism permeated the cultural fabric of Orissa so deeply that it became a key factor in the shaping of the region's history.

But before Shaivism became the dominant faith of the people of Orissa, in the 8th century AD, royal patronage under the Bhaumakaras returned to Mahayana Buddhism, indicating the continuing struggle between the two faiths that eventually ended in the triumph of Shaivism. This era was remarkable for consolidating Orissa in a number of ways, including its geographic territory, religious thought and artistic tradition. During this period, tantrism, which originated as a practice of the Buddhists became a lasting feature of Shaivism. The period witnessed an integration of tantrism, Shaivism, and Mahayana Buddhism that influenced all aspects of Oriya culture from art to architecture to dance. The most compelling evidence of this amalgamation can be seen in the Vaital, Markandeswar, and Sisireswar temples, in the Buddhist *stupas* at the Lalitgiri and Ratnagiri hills, and in the circular hypaethral *yogini* temples of Hirapur which provide sculptural representations of the dance tradition of this historic period.

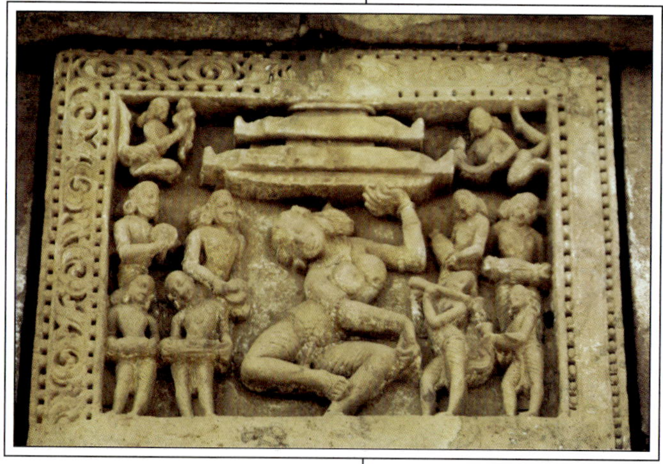

A stone relief depicting a highly stylised presentation of the tribhangi *posture of Odissi.*

In the 10th century AD, the Kesari dynasty had established Shaivism as the single dominant faith. The religion of the royalty gradually became the accepted faith of the people. Shiva worship and the construction of temples dedicated to Lord Shiva took centre stage.

The Kesari temples portrayed various sculptures of dancing gods and humans that indicate the continuation of the Shaivite dancing tradition. But in addition to the sculptural evidence of the dance form, it is believed that the Kesari era was the first to have inscriptional records of a *devadasi* (literally, servant of god) dancing tradition. The *devadasis* were temple servants whose sole duty was to dance at rituals and ceremonies associated with the temple and for the deity within. The earliest record of the *devadasi* tradition in Orissa dates back to the time of the construction of the Brahmeswar Temple by Udyota Kesari, the last king of the Kesari dynasty. The Kesari rule eventually ended some time in the early 11th century.

The Brahmeswar Temple inscription is a landmark in the history of Odissi dance as it chronicles the birth of the temple dancing tradition that would gradually evolve into the Odissi dance of today.

In its first thousand years of existence, the history of the dance tradition of Orissa was synonymous with the political and religious history of the region. From the tolerance and aesthetic awareness of Buddhists to the *yogini* dancers of tantric cults to the glory of Shaivite temple dancing girls, the dance tradition metamorphosed in its physical technique and religious association during each stage of Orissa's early history. Though the Kesari era is celebrated as having established many of the fundamental elements of dance in Orissa, it was not until the Kesari dynasty faded away that the Odissi dance that exists today began to emerge.

When the vacuum created by the decline of the Kesaris was finally filled by the imperial Gangas in the early 11th century, Orissa witnessed the birth of a new religious creed that permanently altered the history of the region—Vaishnavism. Celebrated for their devotion to Lord Vishnu, their construction of the monumental temple of Jagannath at Puri and the Sun Temple at Konark, and their patronage of the *devadasi* dance tradition, the Ganga dynasty revolutionised the entire cultural pattern of Orissa.

A temple in Bhubaneswar.

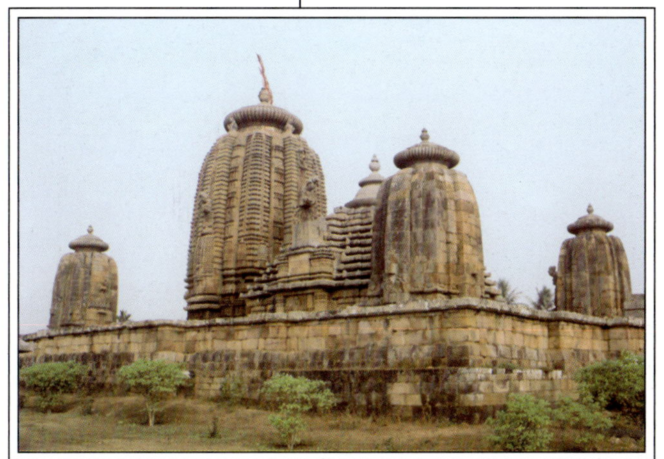

Studies of art and architecture after the Kharavela period strengthen the fact that dance formed a significant theme and essence of Oriya temples. Dance, which is believed to have first appeared during King Kharavela's rule of ancient Orissa around the 1st century BC, experienced immense changes in its physical form, its spiritual character, and its role in society and religion. The character of this divine dance form alternated with Jainism, Buddhism, Shaivism, and Vaishnavism—religions that were dominant at one time or another with the changing dynasties of Kalinga. The encouraging influence of all these religions gave the tradition of dance a distinct sacred character—blending sanctity with beauty, and art with religion, in a humble search for the path to *moksha* or salvation.

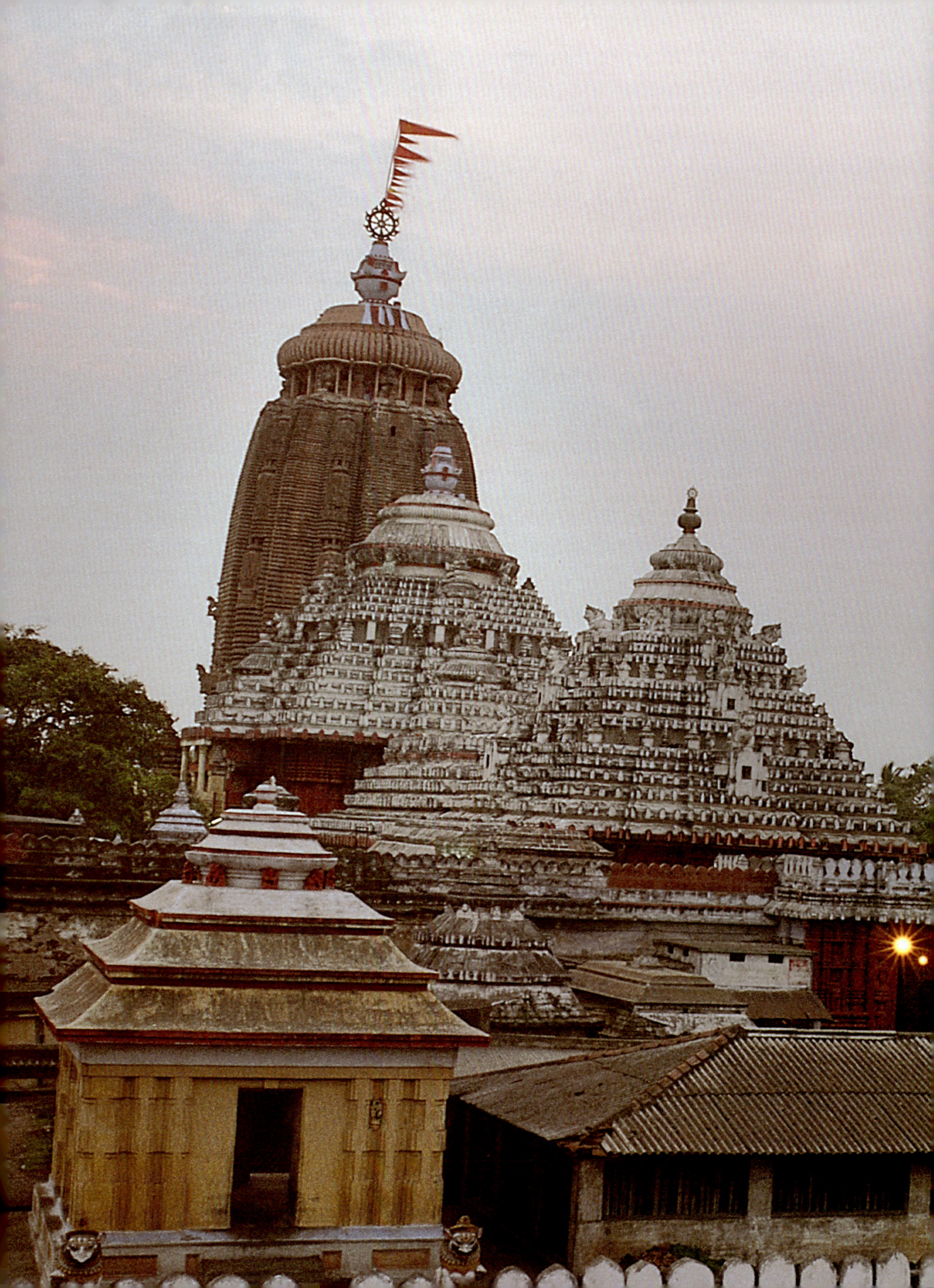

LORD JAGANNATH

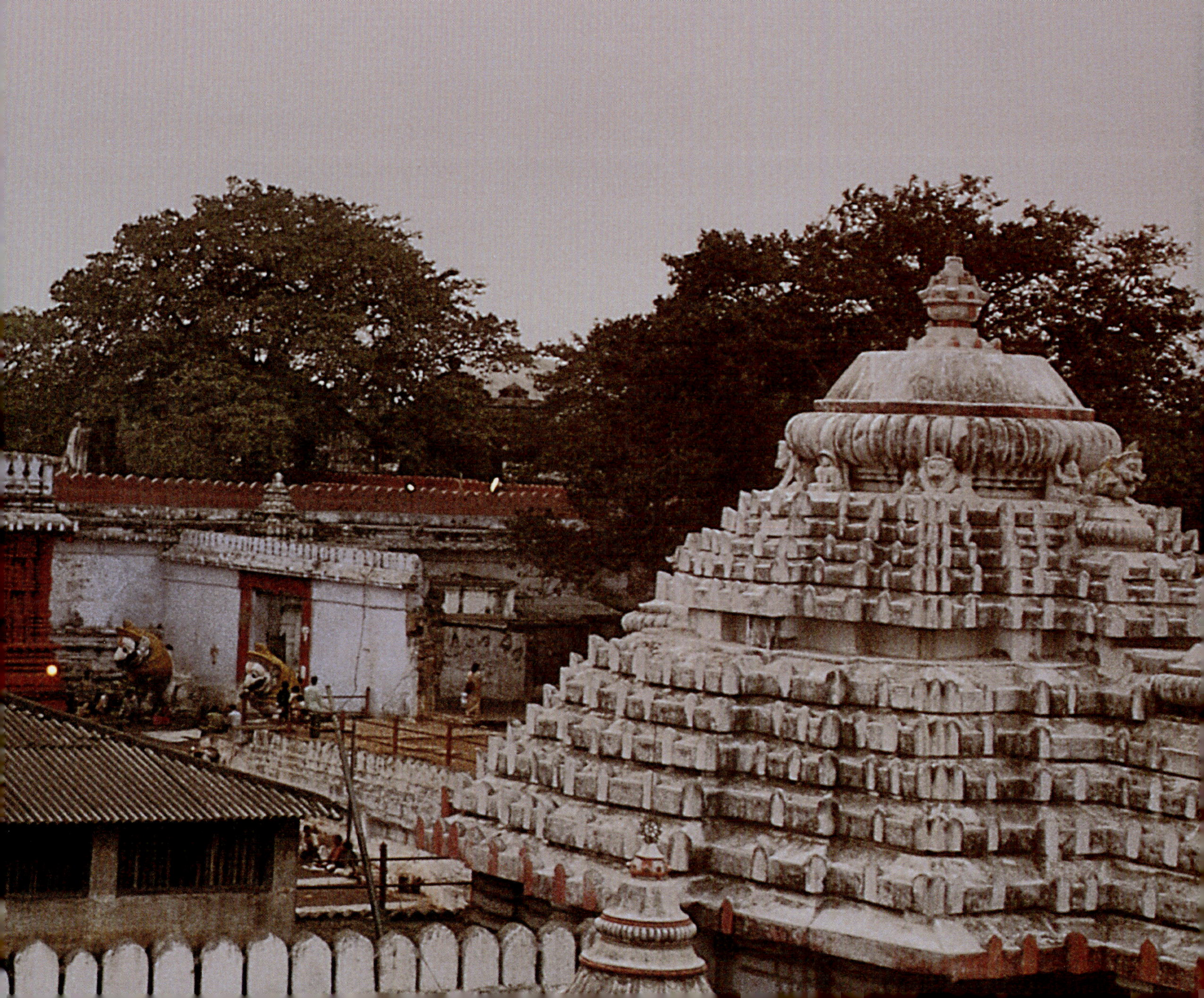

The construction of the monumental Jagannath Temple marked the culmination of a gradual shift in the religious thought in Orissa from Shaivism to Vaishnavism. The art form today known as Odissi is a direct descendant of the temple dance that evolved in the temple of Lord Jagannath at Puri.

The Ganga kings, who were to rule Orissa for nearly three centuries, are best remembered for their devotion to Vaishnavism and the construction of the famous temple of Lord Jagannath at Puri in the 11th century by Anantavarma Chodagangadeva, their first king. During the years of the Ganga rule, the Vaishnavite deity of Jagannath was elevated to the position of the state deity of Orissa. The temple in Puri came to be revered as one of the holiest places of pilgrimage in India and became the centre of culture, religion and artistic tradition in the region. This fact is enhanced by the temple walls adorned with images of the gods and their accompanying celestial dancers, musicians and the various scriptures. In the inner sanctum of this majestic shrine was born the dance of the *mahari.*

Vaishnavism is based on Lord Vishnu and his various *avataras*, or incarnations, in which he is believed to have descended to the earth to save the world from chaos and destruction. Vaishnavism is known to have existed since the time of the *Rig Veda*, a text in which Vishnu is conceived as a

Preceding double spread: A view of the Jagannath Temple complex in pre-dawn light.

Below: An old engraving of the Jagannath Temple.

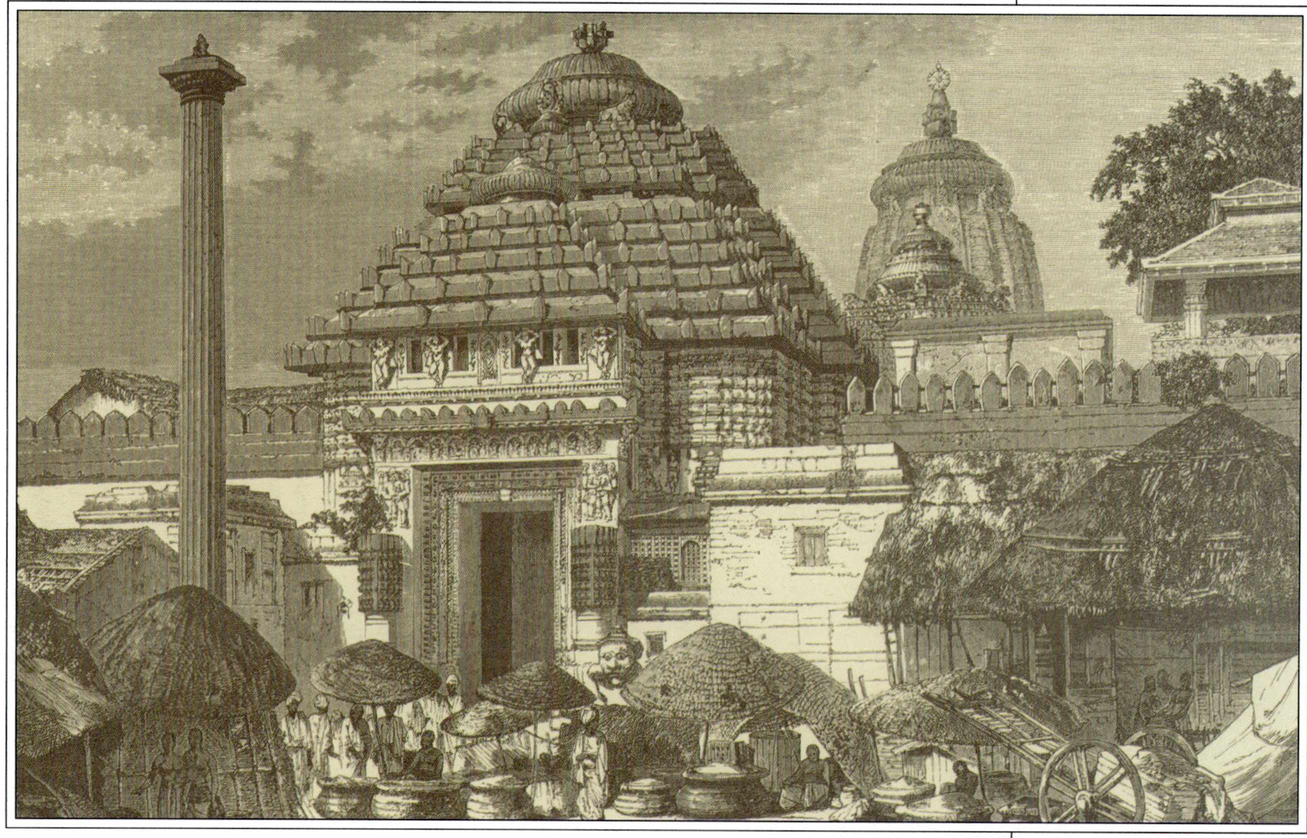

manifestation of the sun. Vaishnavism seems to have first appeared in Orissa around the 7th century AD. For the first time, sculptures of Lord Krishna, one of Vishnu's most popular incarnations, came to be included in temple architecture. Other forms of Lord Vishnu were also worshipped during various stages of Orissa's history, but he seems to have enchanted the most as Lord Jagannath.

There are different traditions in mythology relating to the origin of Lord Jagannath, but perhaps the best loved and most central to Odissi dance is that relating to King Indradyuman and his discovery of the image of Lord Vishnu. King Indradyuman dreamt of the existence of an image of Nilamadhav (the Blue God—another name for Lord Vishnu) in the mountains towards the east. He sent his minister, Vidyapati, to the region where he came across Vishvavasu, the chief of the Savara tribe and a great devotee of Nilamadhav. Vidyapati informed King Indradyuman that he had found the image of Nilamadhav. King Indradyuman then sent an army, which vanquished Vishvavasu and his tribe so that he could acquire the image of Nilamadhav personally. But before the king reached the caves where the deity was, a storm hit, amid which the image of Nilamadhav disappeared. The Blue God no longer appeared to the Savara tribe but revealed his image as a block of timber as if expelled from the ocean on the sand. Again King Indradyuman experienced the same revelation

A depiction of Lord Jagannath, Subhadra and Balabhadra in a traditional palm-leaf drawing of Orissa.

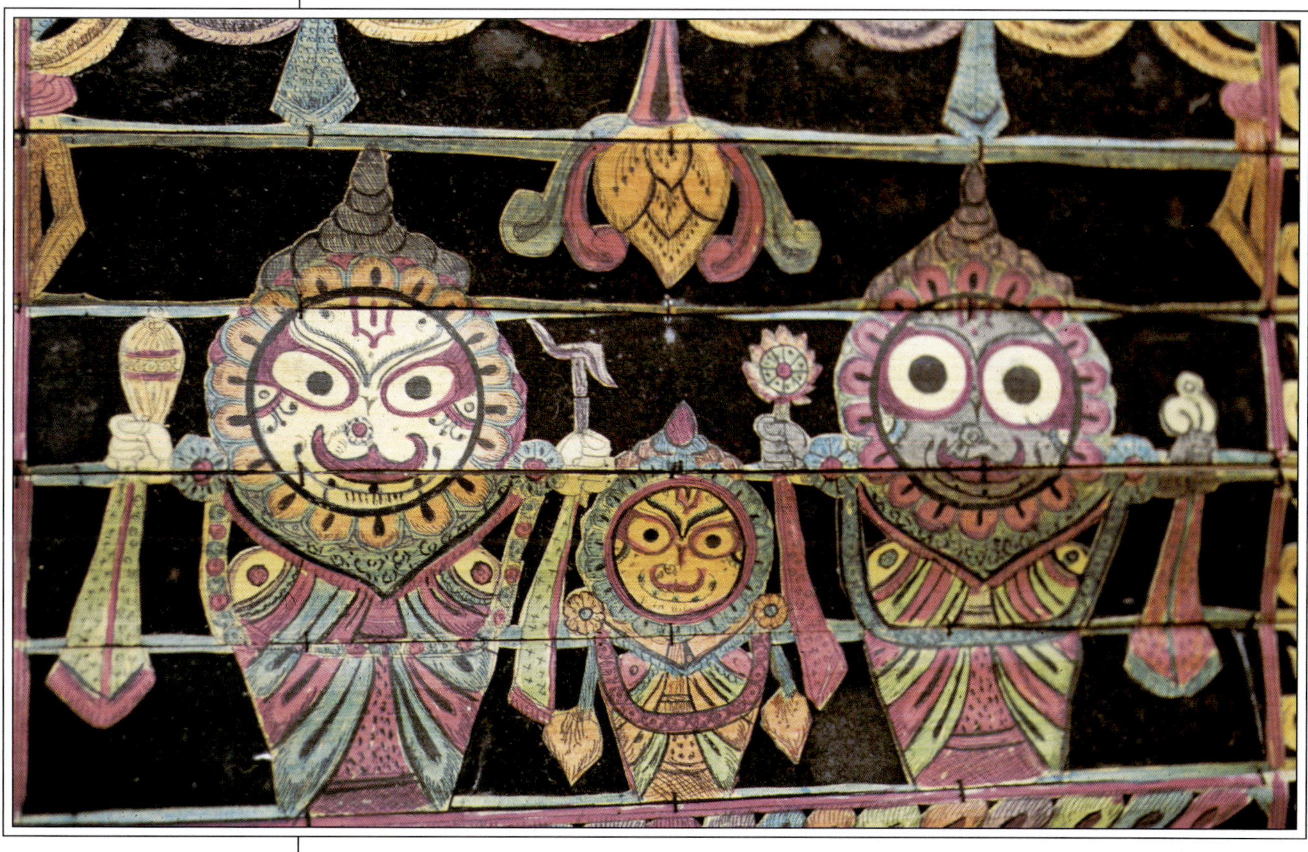

and he brought the log of wood to his palace. He then gathered carpenter-artisans to create an image of Lord Jagannath out of that log. All the carpenters failed to create the image, except one who was believed to be Lord Vishnu Himself. This carpenter's only request was that he should be left undisturbed in the temple for 21 days while he carved the log. The queen, however, in her restlessness and curiosity persuaded the king to open the doors before the promised time. The moment the doors were opened, the carpenter vanished and three incomplete images were found carved into the log. These images, designed from the waist upwards, were of Lord Jagannath, his brother Balabhadra and sister Subhadra. All the three are worshipped till today.

Lord Jagannath is an excellent example of Hindu tribal dichotomy in India, which finally finds its lasting manifestation in the temple in Puri. The existence of former tribals (*daitas*) and Vedic Brahmins amongst its priests is by no means an antithesis, but a splendid regional synthesis of the local and pan-Indian traditions which have integrated the faith and made Puri one of the *Char dhams* or the four most revered shrines of the country.

During the millennium that elapsed between the time of the first appearance of the dance and the construction of the Jagannath Temple, the

Lord Jagannath dominates all festivities of Orissa.

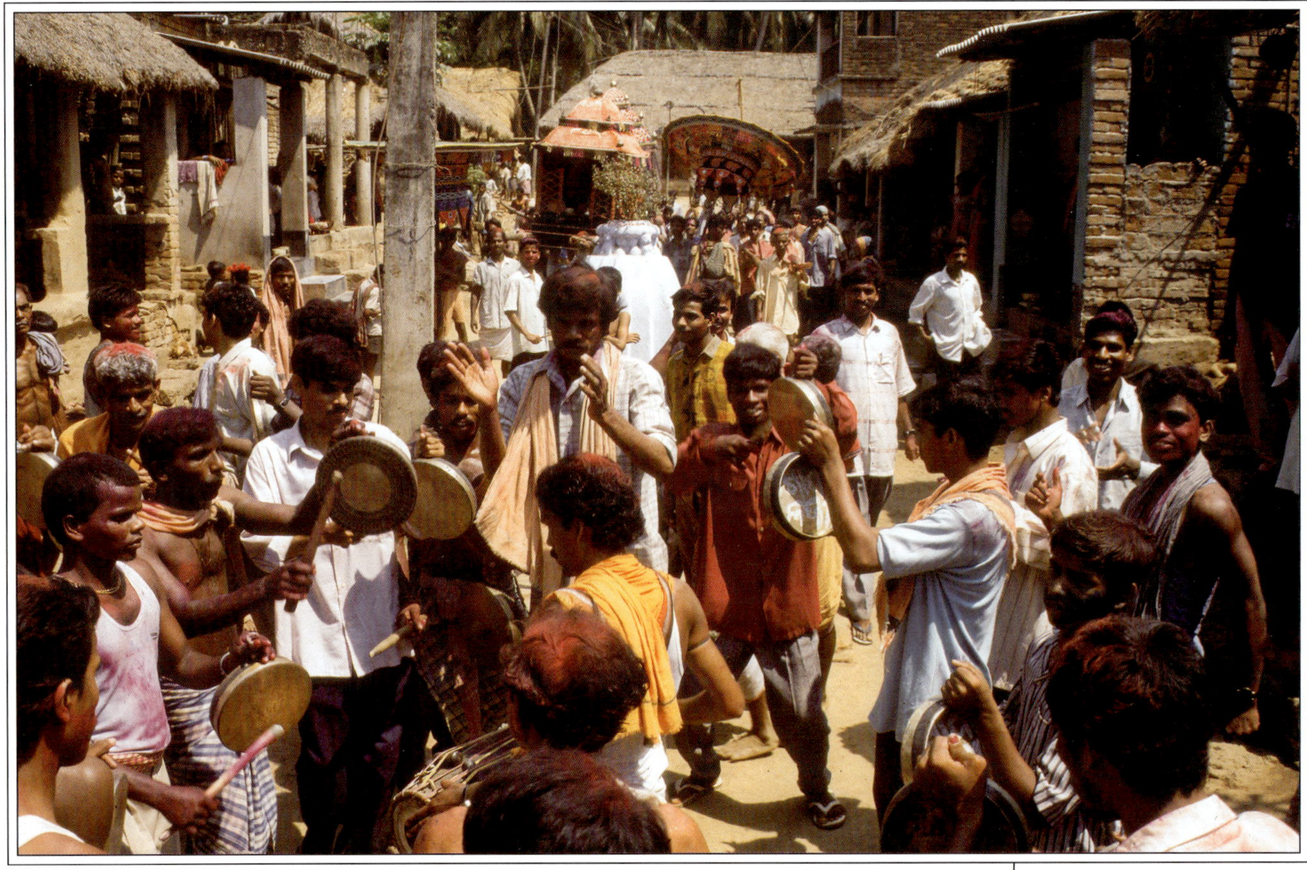

form survived and flourished under the patronage of many of the dynasties that ruled over the region, including the Chedi dynasty (1st to 2nd century BC), the Sailodbhava kings (7th century AD), and the Bhaumakaras (8th century AD). In the 10th and 11th centuries, Orissa experienced an outburst of temple building that began under the Kesari dynasty and reached great heights under the rule of the powerful Gangas. The Ganga kings, are best remembered for their devotion to Vaishnavism and their construction of the famed temple of Lord Jagannath. Though the deity now known as Lord Jagannath, meaning Lord of the World, is most commonly worshipped as a Vaishnavite deity, the origins of the god actually represent an amalgamation of religious traditions, including local tribal beliefs, Jainism, Buddhism, Shaivism, *tantrism* and, of course, Vaishnavism.

The accession of Chodagangadeva, who was perhaps the greatest monarch of the Ganga dynasty, in 1077 AD marked a turning point in the religious history of Orissa. Influenced by the teachings of the Vaishnavite philosopher, Ramanuja, and keenly aware of the growing popularity of the Jagannath cult, Chodagangadeva made a politically motivated decision to consolidate his rule by appealing to the religious interests of his people. His patronage of Vaishnavism was not only the singular most significant act of the Ganga rule but also an important aspect of the history of Orissa, for it established the historical foundation of what was to be the greatest socio-political-religious force the region had ever experienced.

Following double spread: A portrayal of Jayadeva singing and Padmavati dancing.

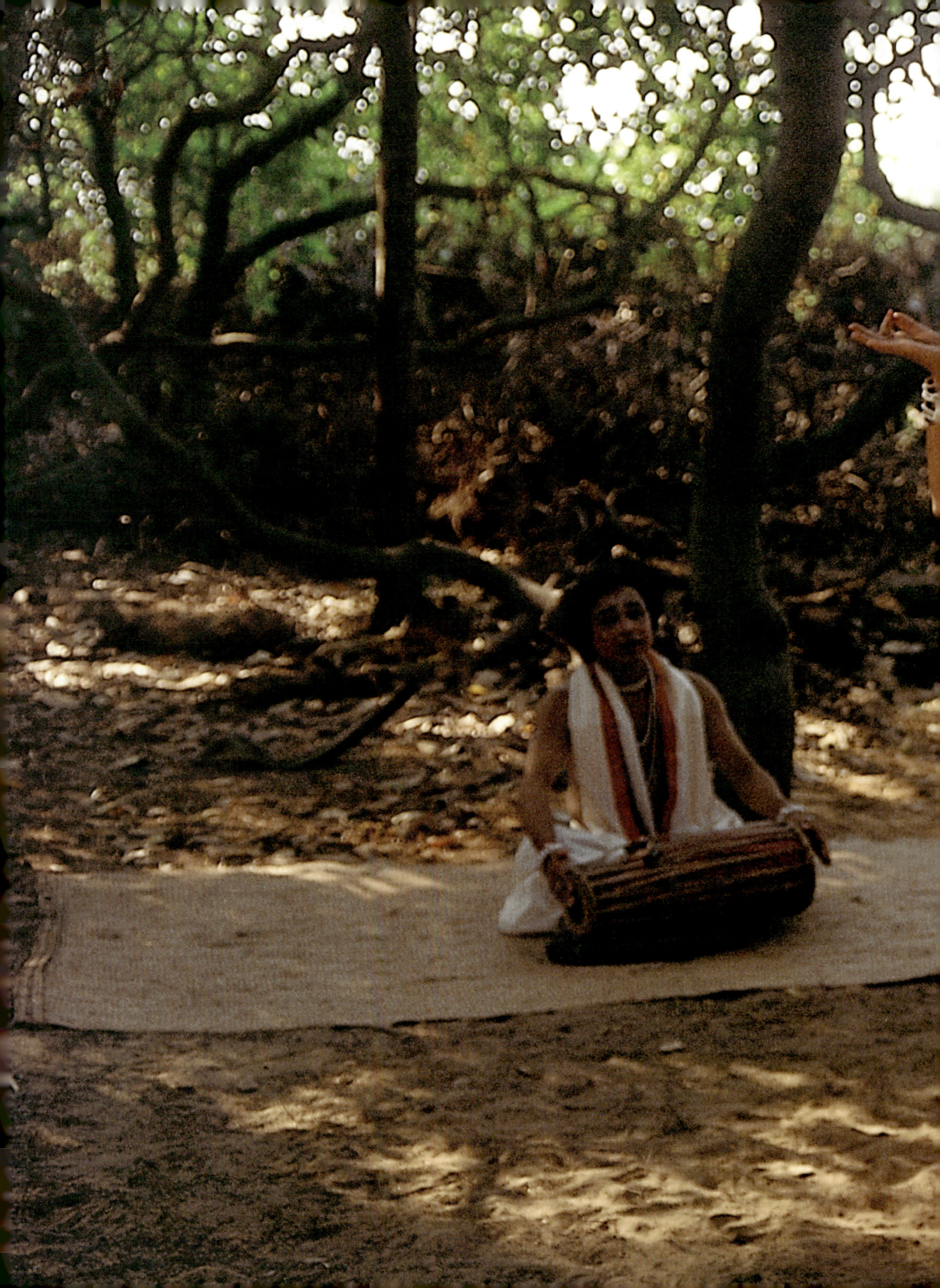

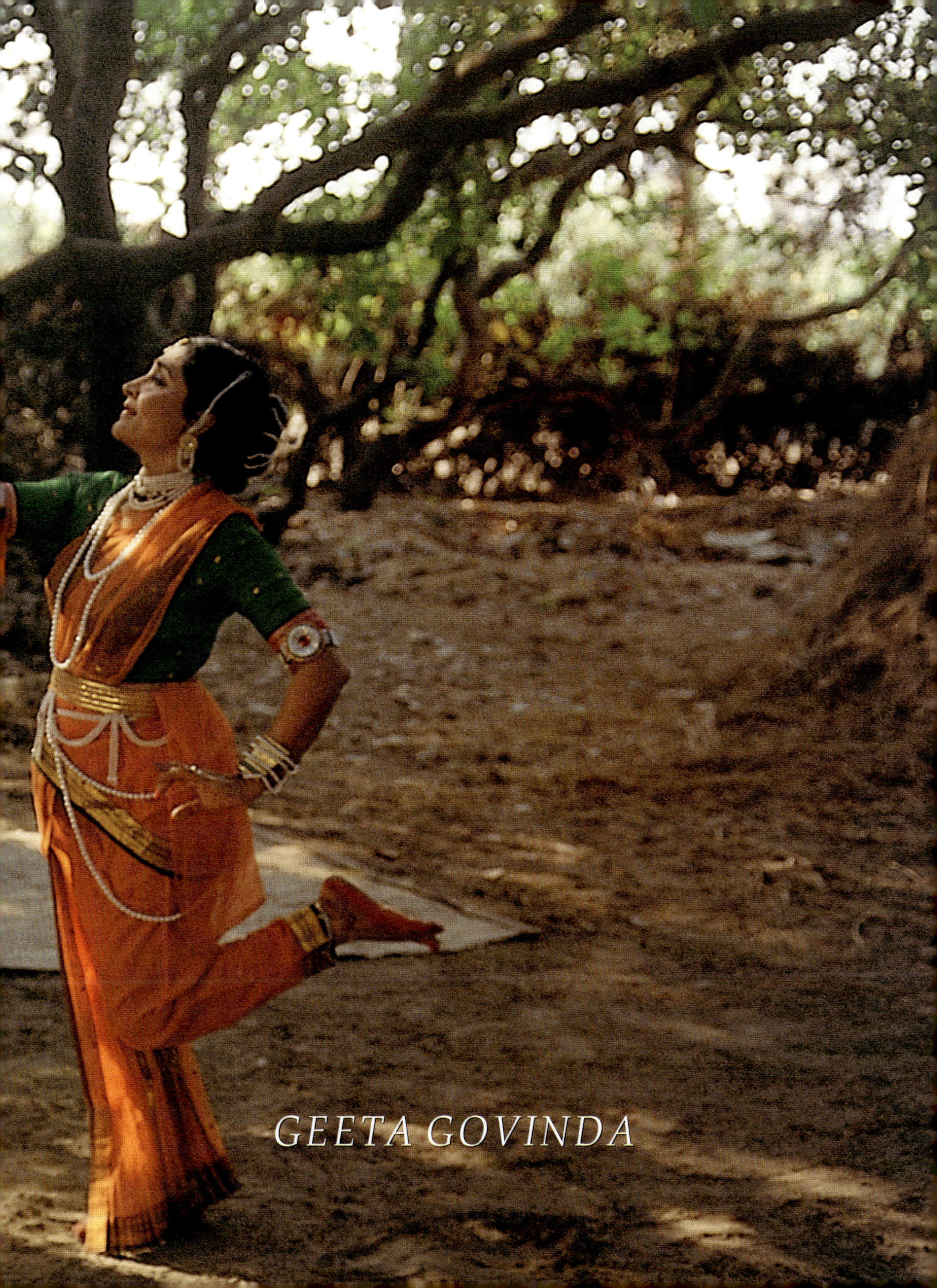

GEETA GOVINDA

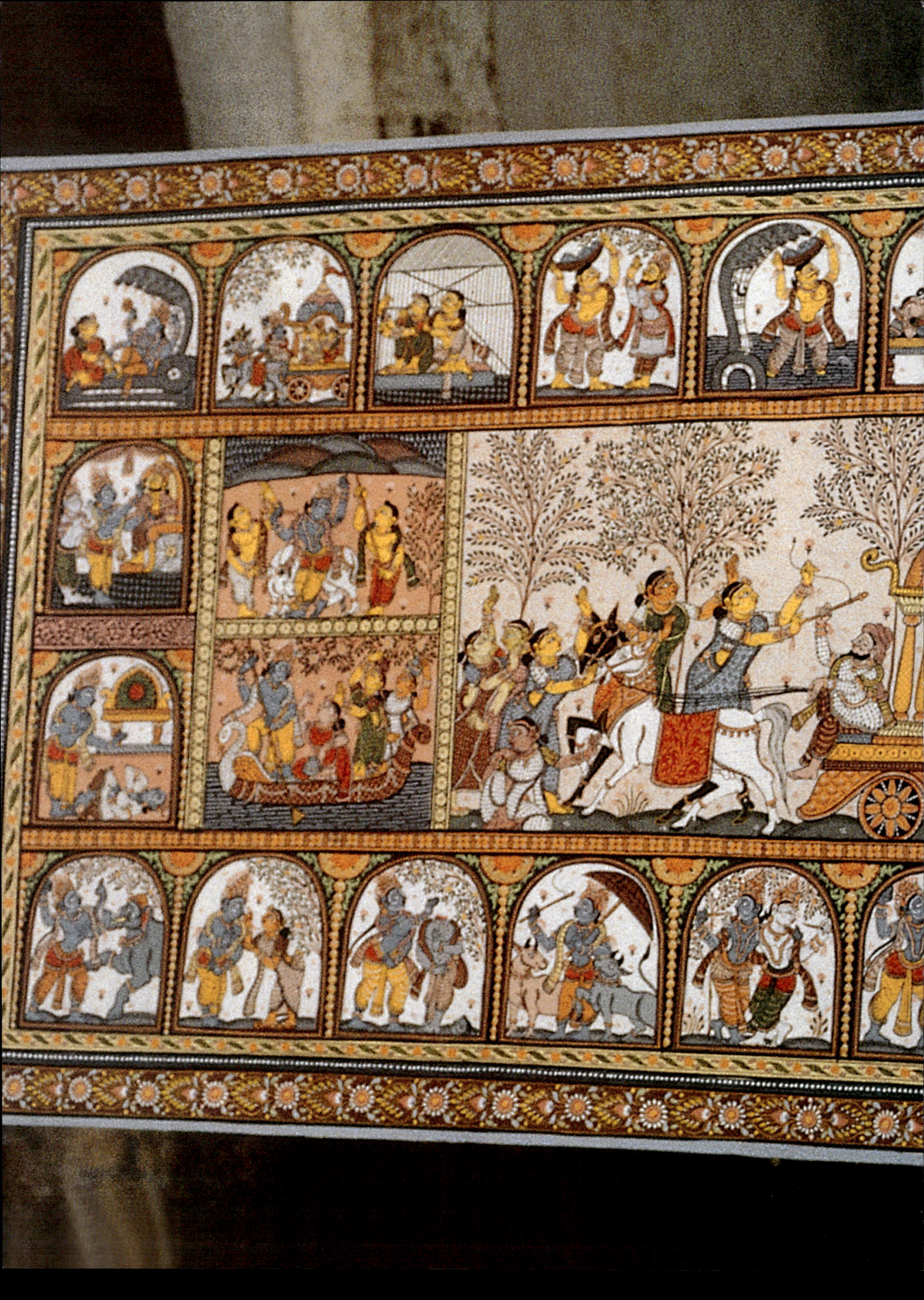

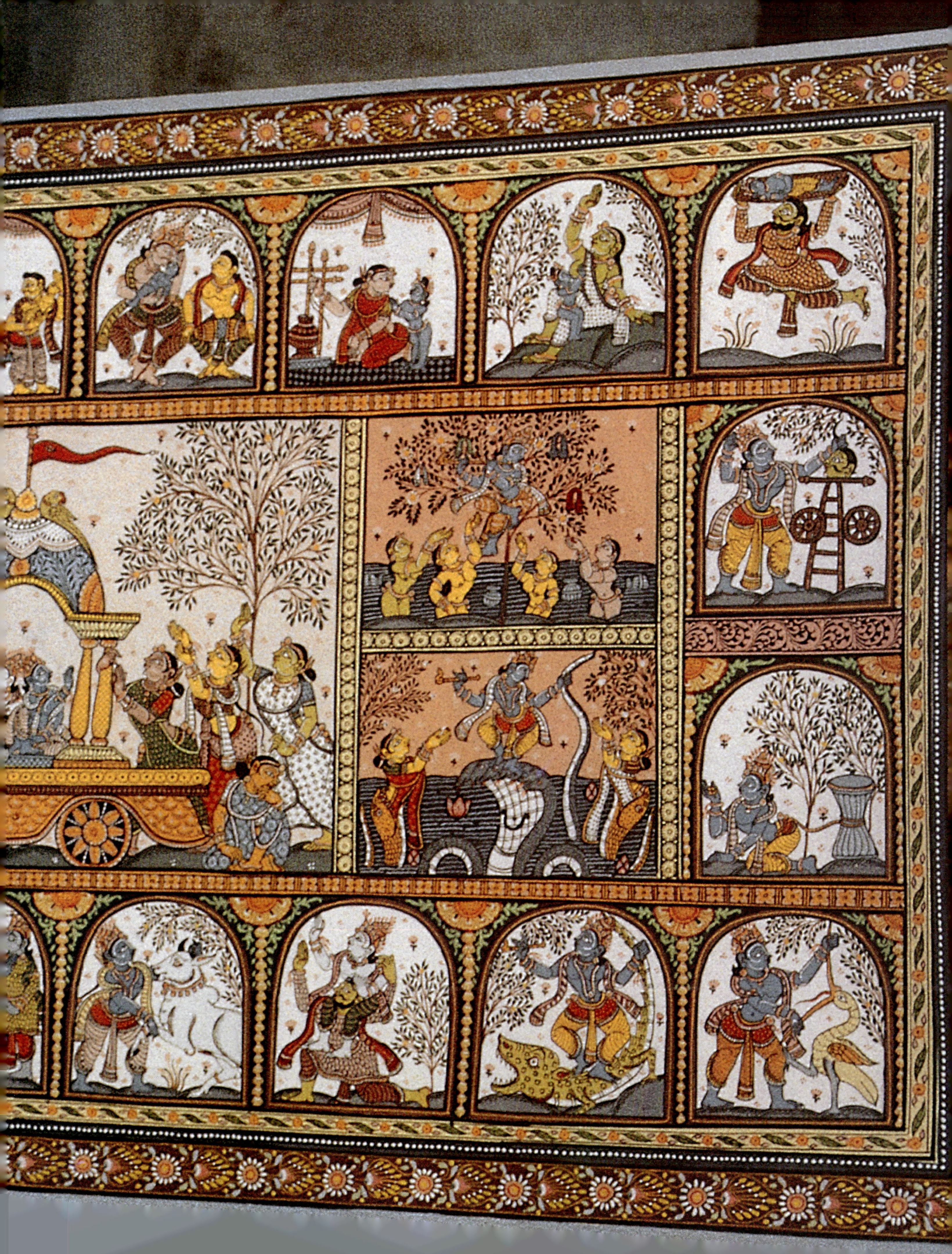

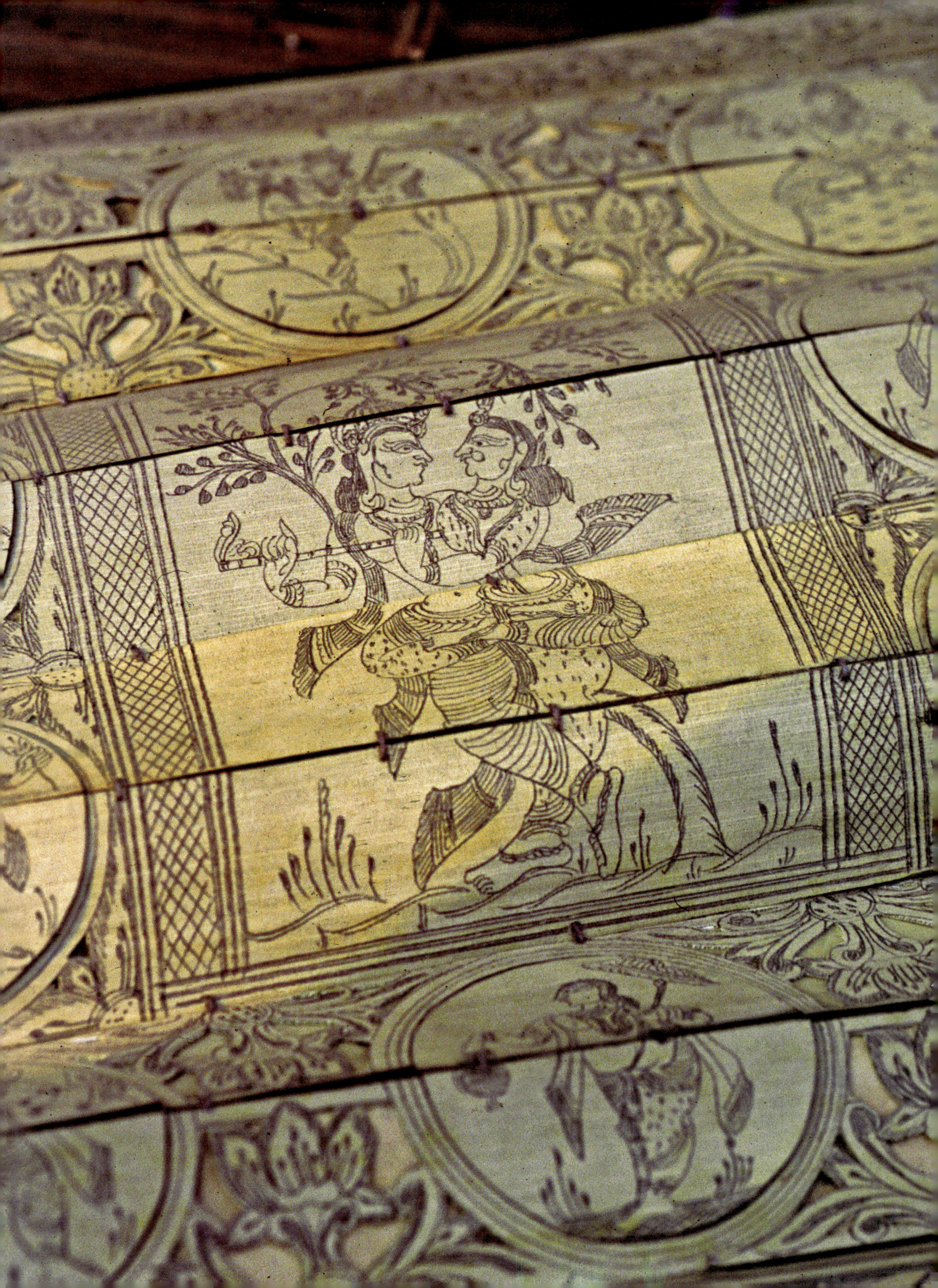

The *Geeta Govinda,* written in Sanskrit by the saint poet Sri Jayadeva in the 12th century, occupies a special place in the history of Indian literature and dance. A celebration of the love between Lord Krishna and his beloved Radha, the *Geeta Govinda* is often interpreted as an allegory of a devotee's love for the Lord. It has come to be acknowledged as the supreme illustration of romantic poetry that enhances the Indian tradition and is the culmination of the essence of the Sanskrit poetic traditions. Descriptive of unmatched romance and devotion, it is sung, chanted, and performed even today, eight centuries after it was composed.

It is said that to inspire Jayadeva to write the *Geeta Govinda,* the Lord introduced the love of Padmavati, believed to have been a *mahari* in the temple of Jagannath, as a wife into his life. The life and history of Jayadeva are set in the village of Kenduvilvasasana or Kendulisasana in Puri, and the legends narrate the significance of the poet and the poem to the history of both devotion to Lord Jagannath as well as the *mahari* tradition. Padmavati, who is described as 'a paragon of beauty, a storehouse of wisdom, an ideal wife and an ardent devotee of Krishna', taught Jayadeva the way of human love that inspired his masterpiece, the *Geeta Govinda*. Theirs is believed to be an ideal physical union because of their marriage and an ideal spiritual union because of their collective

Preceding double spread: Patachitra *depicting the heroic stories of Krishna in Vrindavan.*

Left: Radha and Krishna in a dance of joy.

Below: A sculpture of Krishna as a child.

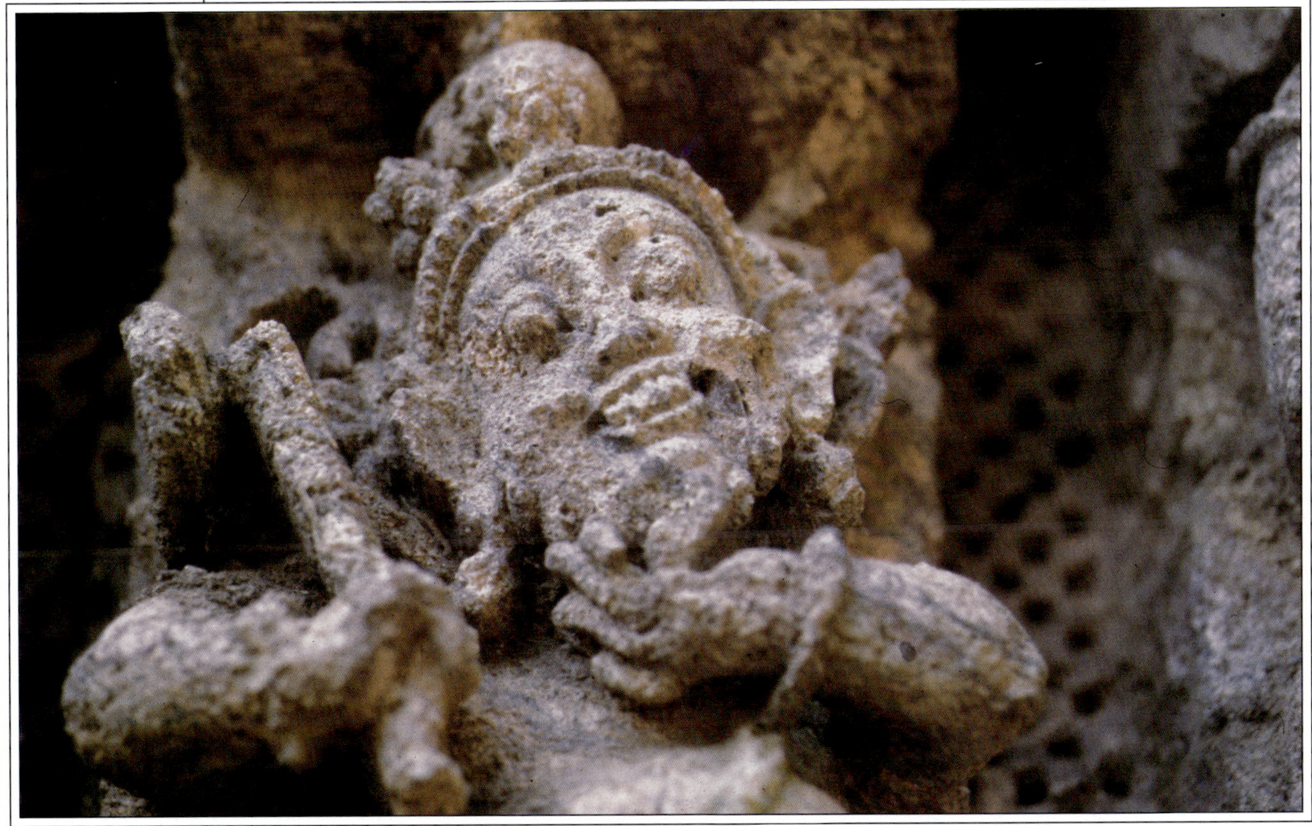

devotion to Krishna—Jayadeva's through his verse and Padmavati's through her dance.

One of the legends about the composition of the *Geeta Govinda* suggests that Lord Krishna appeared in the guise of a poet and completed the last couplet, when Jayadeva was confronted by a writer's block. Seeing Jayadeva's frustration, Padmavati suggested that he revive his spirits with a bath in the river and then try to finish the couplet. He went to bathe and, in the meantime, Krishna appeared in the guise of the poet and started penning down from where Jayadeva had left off. He wrote:

स्मरगरलखण्डनं मम शिरसि मण्डनं देहि पदपल्लवमुदारम्।
ज्वलति मयि दारुणो मदनकदनारुणो हरतु तदुपाहितविकारम्।।

Smargaralakhandana mama shirasi mandana dehi padapallavmudaram I
Jyolati mayi daruno madankadanaruno haratu tadupahitavikaram II

O Radha, place the noble sprout of your foot as an ornament upon my head, for it dispels the poison of love.

These are the famous lines which Lord Krishna is believed to have helped create. Lovingly he also ate the food prepared by Padmavati. When Jayadeva returned, both of them realised that they had received the divine grace of Krishna.

The description of the physical beauty of men, women and Nature in the *Geeta Govinda* is highly aesthetic and refined, for Radha and Krishna have been treated as symbols of ideal beauty.

The images of Jayadeva are not only richly nuanced but also interlinked. 'In Jayadeva's hands, the love of Radha and Krishna is not merely the throbbing emotion of the lover and the beloved, but equally the sap that flows through lotus flowers and mango blossoms; the song of Govinda resonates not only in fragrant bowers but also in the cry of the cuckoo; the whisper of their joyous dalliance is shared by the bees that swarm the *bakula* trees; when the lovers are overcome by passion, they are not alone for the *tamala* tree garlanded with fresh leaves is equally overcome by the passion of musk; and the intoxication of spring through the fragrance of the *madhavika* flowers is not only for Radha and Krishna but also produces infatuation even in the minds of sages. It is an enchanted world that Jayadeva creates, for these richly evocative images pulsate in a symphony of colours'. (*The Flute and the Lotus*)

Jayadeva introduced for the first time *raga* and *tala* (rhythm) into the verses of the *Geeta Govinda*, which is also the first exposition of *giti kavya*, or lyrical poetry, in Sanskrit literature. It is interesting to note that the entire *Geeta Govinda* is presumably composed for dance and, from the time of Jayadeva till the present time, it is the favourite theme of dancers.

There are many legends that lead to the belief that Lord Jagannath had a great love for the *Geeta Govinda* and was always present wherever it was sung. It is recorded in the *Madala Panji*, the daily chronicle of the Jagannath Temple that Kavi Narasimbh Deva (1278-1309) introduced the *Geeta Govinda* for the first time in the temple. And in the 15th century under the guidance of Ray Ramanada, Raja Prataparudradeva ordered singing and dancing of the *Geeta Govinda* to be mandatory in the Jagannath Temple. The *Geeta Govinda seva* (service) was performed in the Jagannath Temple by the *maharis*. It was mandatory that in the night (bed-time) worship of the deity, songs from the *Geeta Govinda* were sung along with the dance by the *maharis* to put the God to bed.

By the 15th century, the *Geeta Govinda* was sufficiently popular in Puri to be incorporated into the ritual of the Jagannnath Temple. An inscription on the left of the Jayavijaya doorway, written in Oriya and dated 1499 AD, prescribes the performance of the *Geeta Govinda* ritual in the temple. While established traditions of commentary and manuscripts exist in every part of India, Orissa is probably the largest repository of palm-leaf manuscripts of the *Geeta Govinda*.

Although the poem and the poet originated in eastern India in the 12th century and remained most popular there, it spread throughout the sub-continent in the centuries following its composition, transcended many barriers as it has been translated in more than a hundred languages across the world.

The *Geeta Govinda* has a special place in the temples of Orissa and its lyrics are venerated and sung throughout the state. It influenced Sanskrit literature of the time and strongly impacted art and culture too. It has dominated music, dance, drama, painting, sculpture, literature with *Bhakti* or devotion as the central theme. Even today, the songs of the *Geeta Govinda* are sung in the Jagannath Temple and the verses are visually enacted by the present-day Odissi dancers. It is not a surprise that Odissi and the *Geeta Govinda* are synonymous with each other.

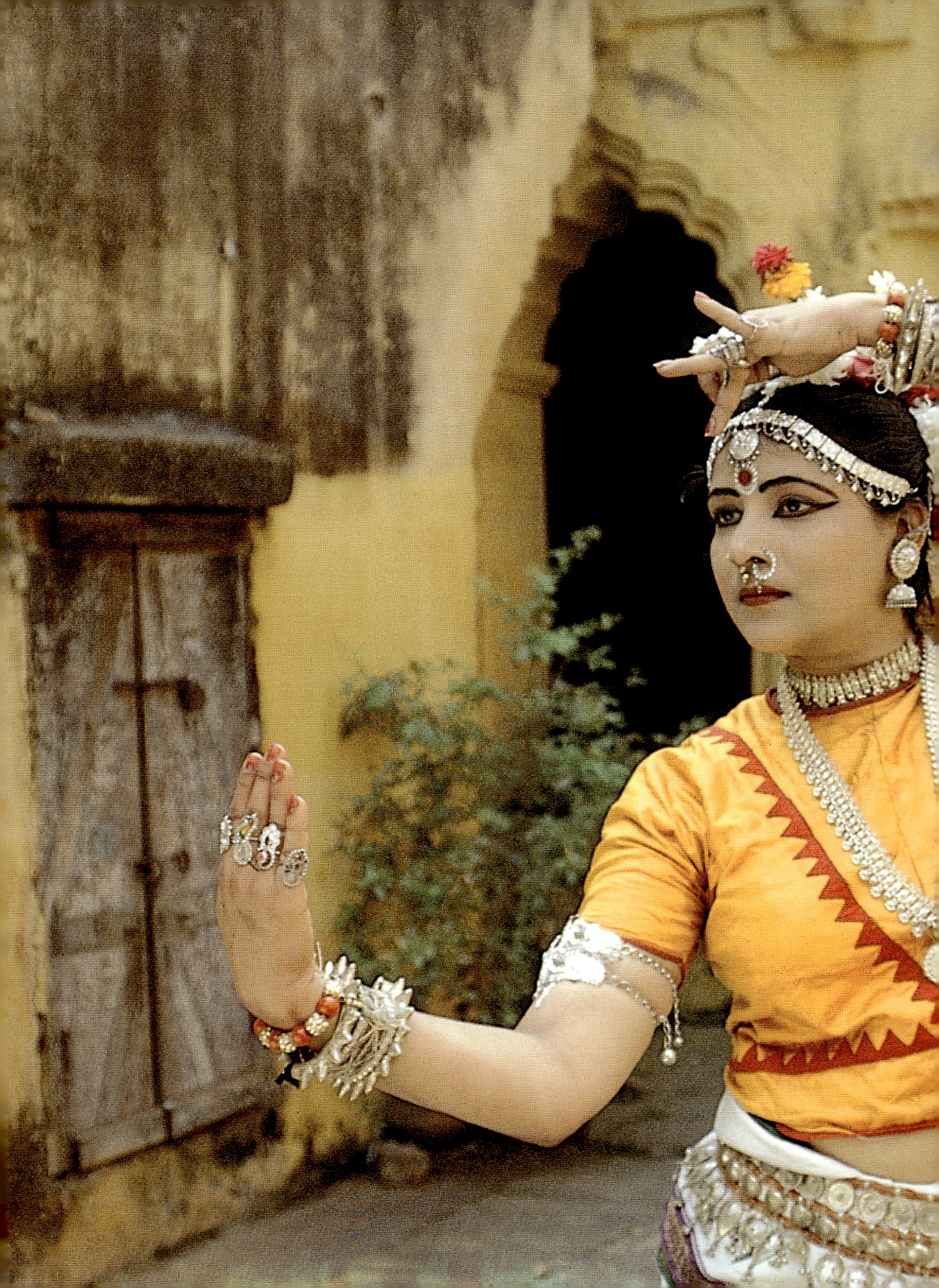

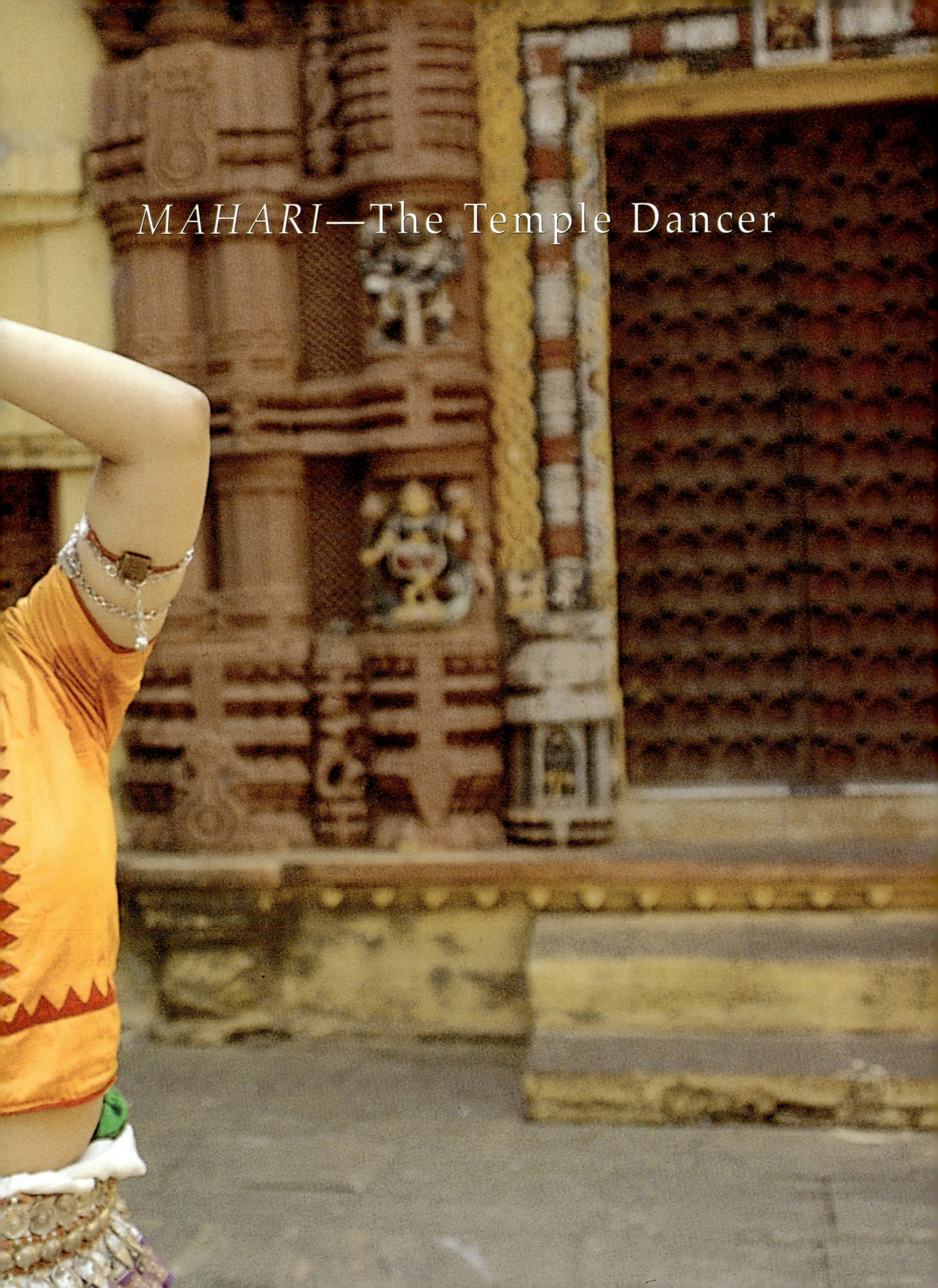

MAHARI—The Temple Dancer

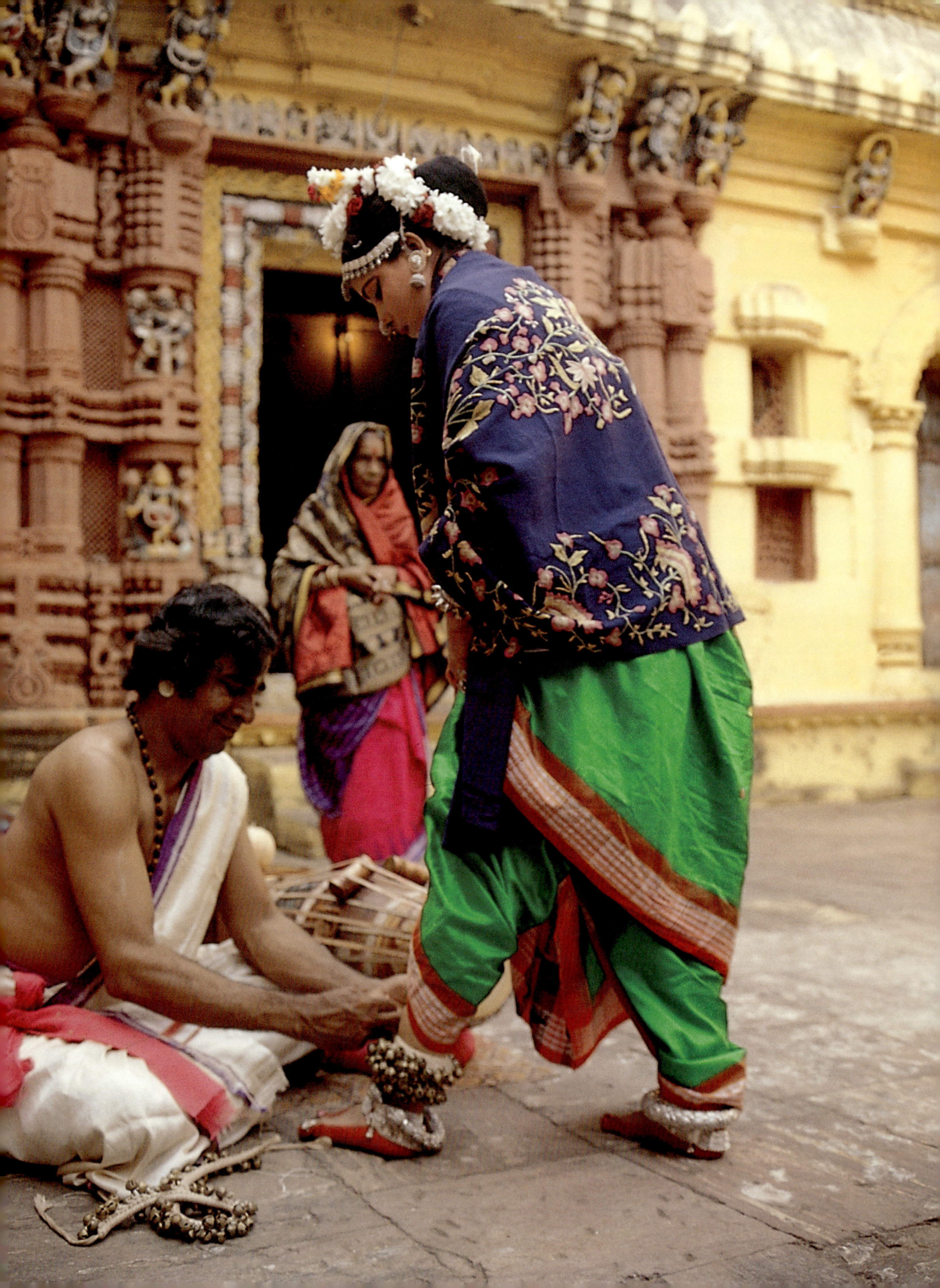

The seat of religion and culture in Orissa, the Jagannath Temple, was also the birthplace of the *mahari* dance tradition. Inscriptions from the 11th century, during the reign of King Anantavarma Chodagangadeva, reveal that the king was a learned man, proficient in the *Vedas* and not only a patron but also a master of the fine arts. The *Madala Panji*, indicates that when the construction of the Jagannath Temple was completed, the king appointed a new class of temple servants known as *maharis*, or temple dancers. The chronicle, maintained daily for several centuries in the temple, gives an elaborate account of their duties and status.

Maharis were women who were 'married' to Lord Jagannath. The marriage ceremony included rituals where the girl, adorned with new clothes and fine jewels, applied *tilak* and sandalwood paste on the forehead. The priest tied one end of Lord Jagannath's clothing around the *mahari's* head in a simple ceremony and initiated her into the *mahari* tradition.

Most often dedicated to the temples at an early age, new *maharis* were either young girls offered to the temple by their families or adopted by the dancers already serving. Once initiated into temple life, young *maharis* learned the arts of music and dance and were educated and groomed accordingly.

Preceding double spread: A mahari *dancer depicting* darpani *with one hand and* tilak *with the other.*

Left: A guru tying ghungroos to a dancer of the mahari *style while the last living* mahari *Shashimoni looks on.*

Below: A mahari *dancer in* abhinaya *pose.*

Following double spread: A mahari *dancer in a charming pose in front of a* historical *math.*

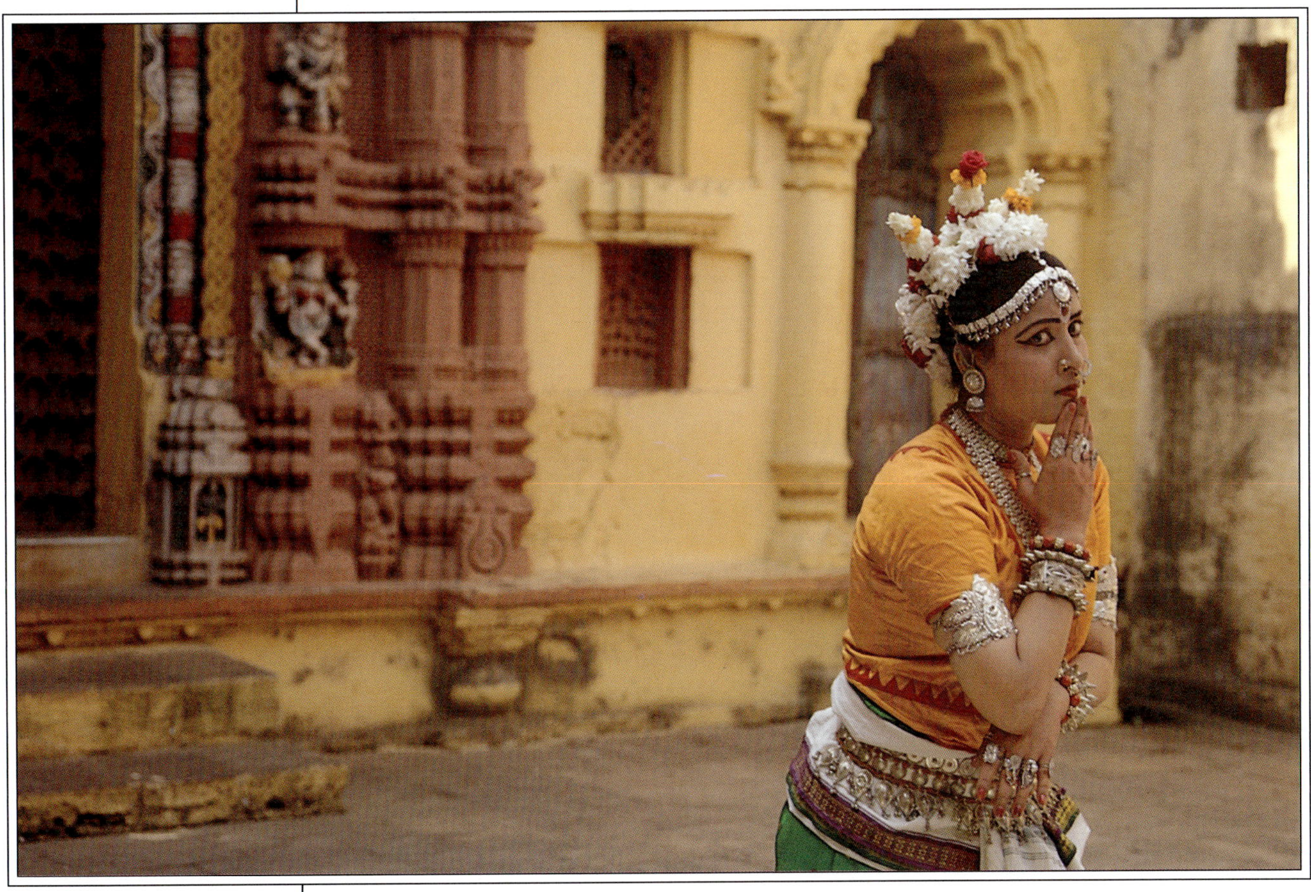

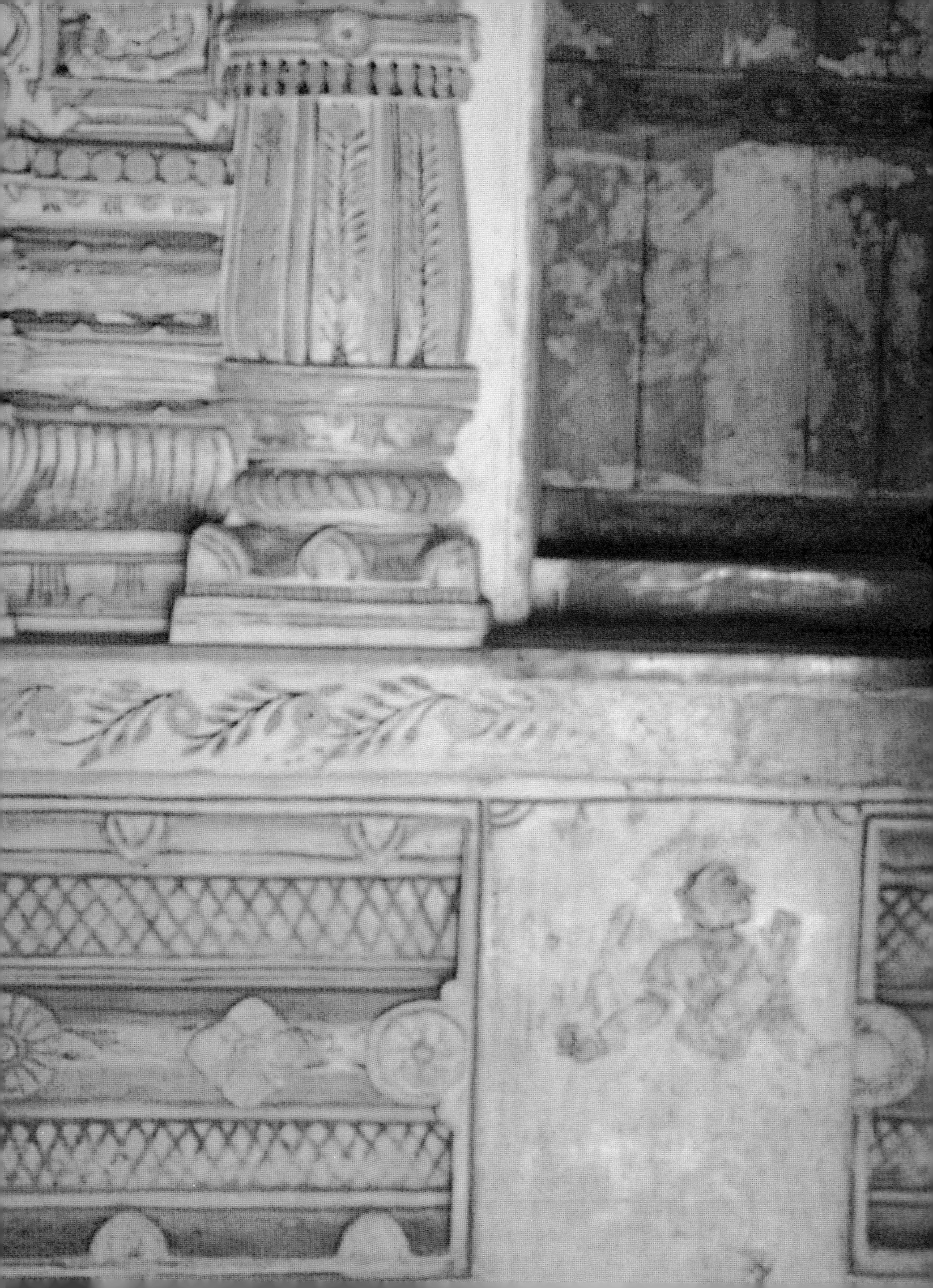

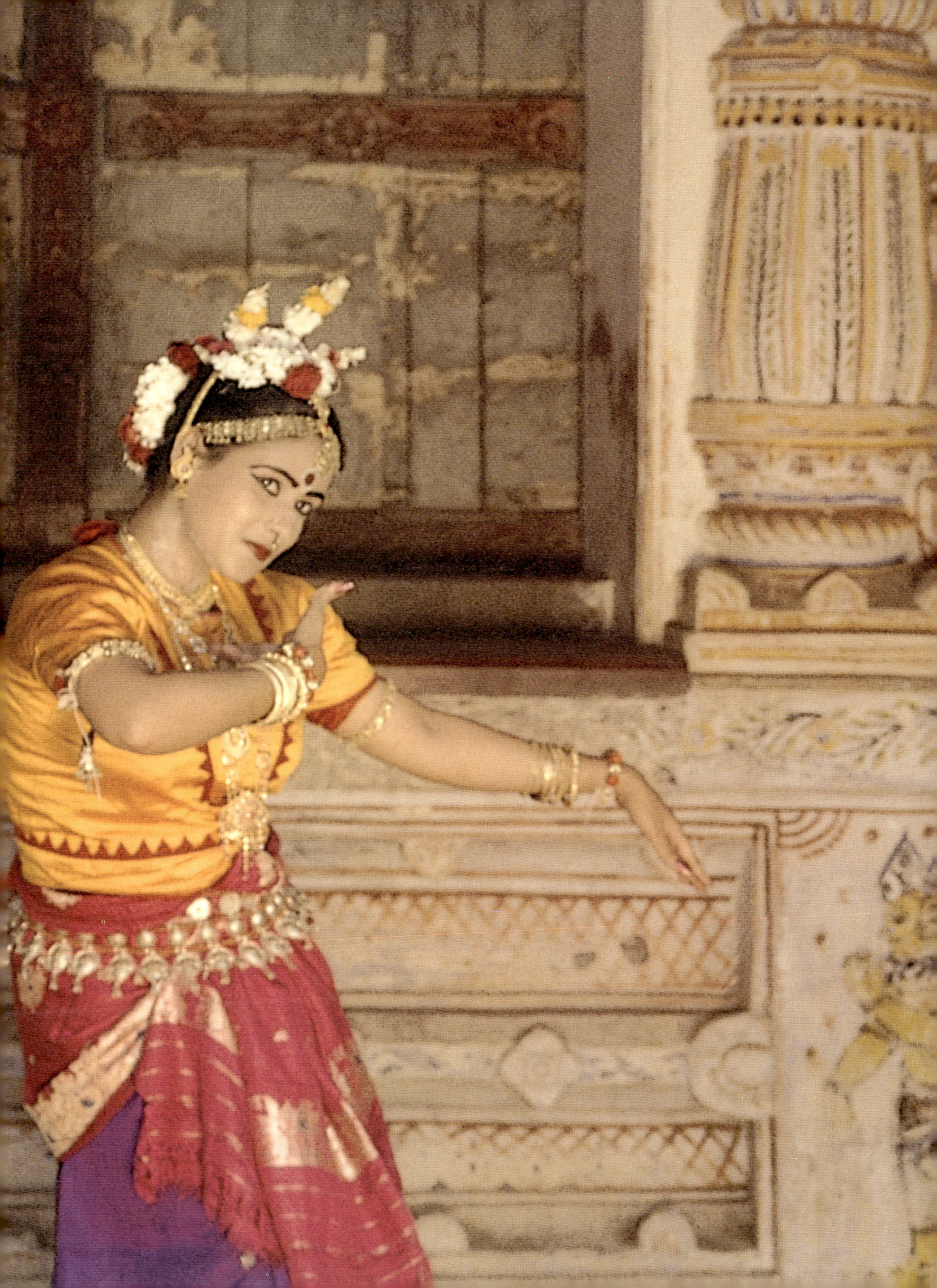

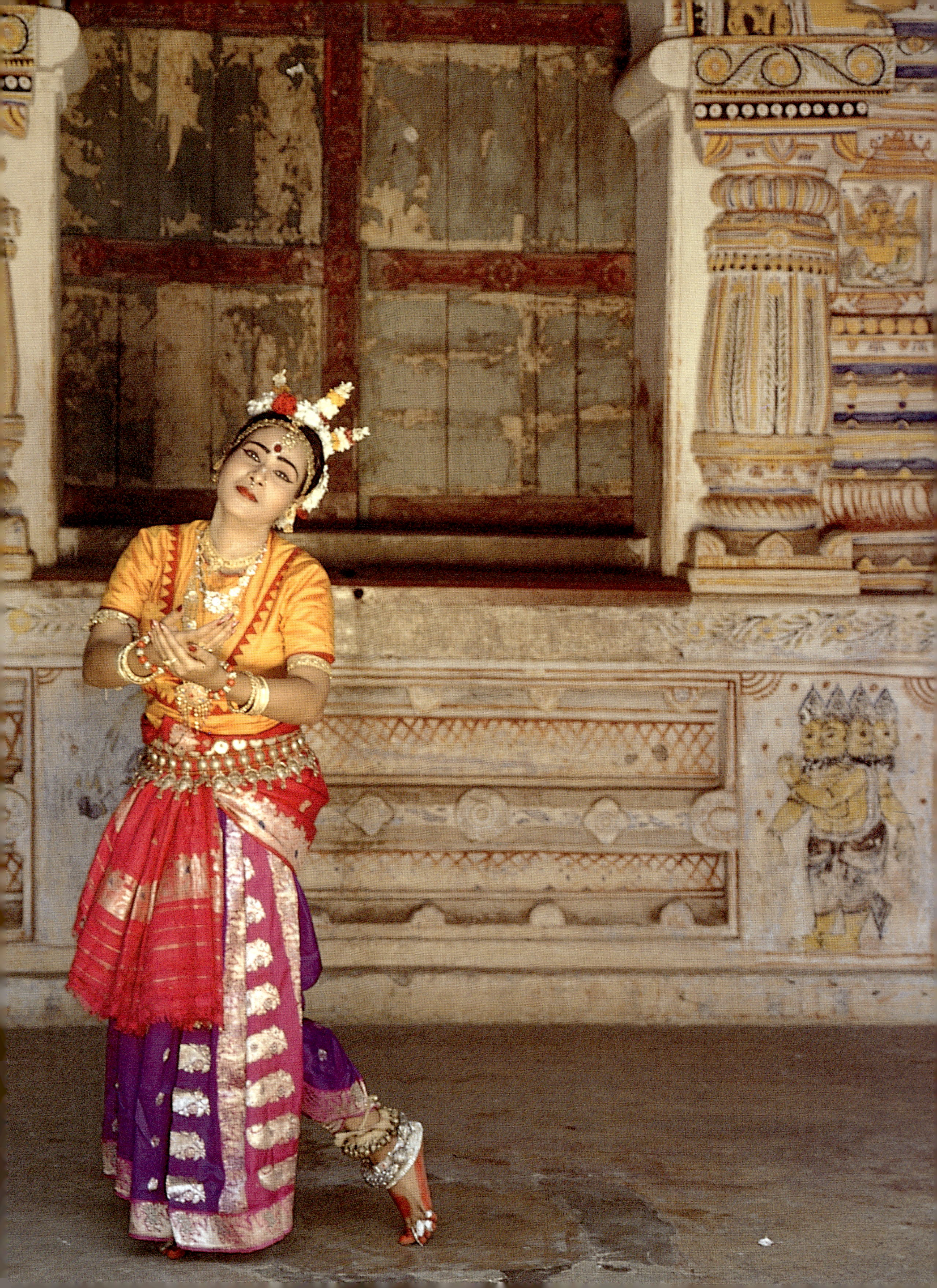

Maharis were divided into several groups according to their services. The dancing girls were known as *nachunis;* singers of the inner apartment were called *bhitara gaunis;* singers who sang outside the temple were called *bahara gaunis;* those whose duty was to fan the lord were called *gaudasanis*. The accompanists—*veenakaras*, the *veena* players, and *madelas*, the *mardala (drum)* players—were males.

Seven streets were built near the temple and each of these was allocated to temple servants belonging to different services in the temple. One of these streets was allotted to the *maharis* and is still known as *mahari palli*. It is also known as *anga alasa patna*. The king appointed officers named *mina nayak* and *sahi nayak* to regulate the services of the *maharis* and provided them sufficient security and stability. The *maharis* were also provided with maintenance, residence and regular income.

The first day of the *mahari* dance training was considered sacred and included a special ceremony with offerings of music and flowers to God and to the dance teacher, or *guru*. Once the girl was proficient in the arts of music and dance, she would begin performing the daily rituals of the temple, which included the morning dance offering, called *sakala dhupa*, the evening ritual of singing, called *sandhya dhupa*, and the bed-time dance, called *bada sringar.*

Although mostly confined to the inner sanctums of the temple, where only high priests or the *rajgurus* were allowed, the *maharis* alone were allowed to dance and sing for Lord Jagannath exclusively. However, when the Jagannath icon was carried through the streets for various festivals, such as the *Chandan Yatra, Ratha Yatra*, and *Jhoolan Yatra*, the *maharis* were allowed to perform their devotional dances for all to see.

Their marriage to the Lord meant that they could never be widowed, and so the *maharis* were considered auspicious and lucky. Educated and cultured, refined and devoted, the *maharis* were cherished and honoured by all.

With the support of the Ganga dynasty, the *maharis* enjoyed high status and prosperity and were greatly encouraged in their art. The patronage of the *mahari* dance tradition and the devotion to Lord Jagannath that developed during the reign of the Ganga dynasty continued till the reign of the Gajapati kings who made enormous contributions to the preservation of the temple in Puri and all its devoted servants, including the *maharis*. Inscriptions referring to the art of the temple dancers are found on nearly all the temples of the Ganga era.

Raja Purushottamdeva of the Suryavansh (solar dynasty), who reigned from 1467 to 1497, was a devotee of Lord Jagannath and a benevolent ruler. A poet and learned man himself, he took keen interest in the transmission of art

Left: A mahari *dancer in an emotional* abhinaya.

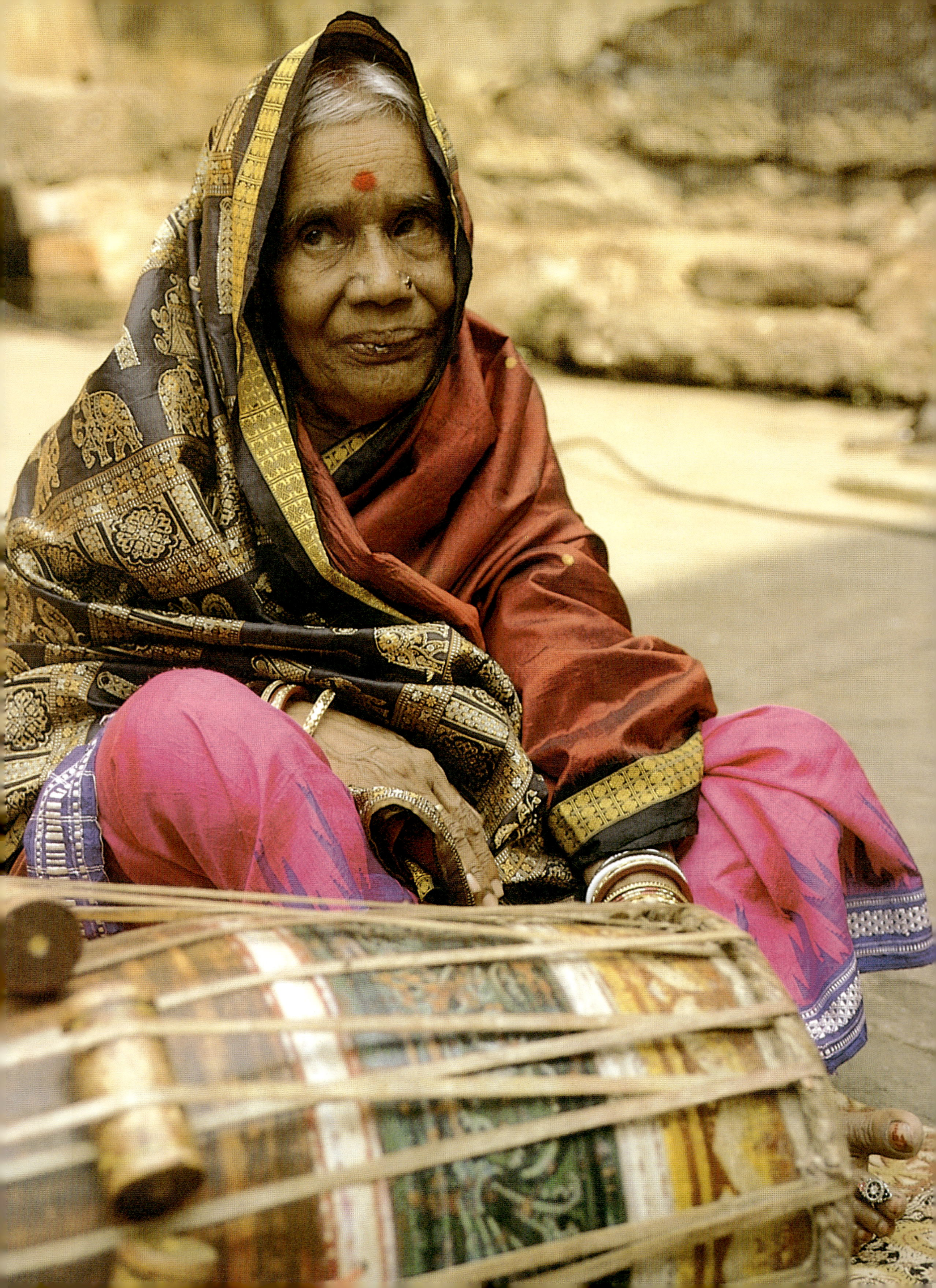

and culture. In fact, there is a popular legend among the people of Orissa about how Purushottamdeva's wife, Padmavati, actually offered herself as a *mahari* to the temple of Lord Jagannath. This legend has immensely influenced Oriya literature and painting, and shows that the *maharis* were held in high esteem and that women of even the royal family considered it an honour to serve the Lord as dancing girls.

In the 15th century, the Gajapati king, Prataparudradeva made singing and dancing of the *Geeta Govinda* mandatory in the Jagannath Temple. His Governor, Ray Ramanada, under the influence of Chaitanya Mahaprabhu, became a devout Vaishnava. He was also a scholar, poet, dramatist, musician and exponent of dance. He introduced *abhinaya*—expression in the dance of the *maharis*—and taught them singing and dancing of the *Geeta Govinda*, which ultimately became an integral part of Odissi dance. The addition of Jayadeva's poem to the repertoire of the *maharis* added to the wealth of knowledge, talent, and refinement that these dancers already possessed.

In 1568, the Afghans started attacking and invading Orissa. These invasions caused major destruction in the Jagannath Temple and its services, and destroyed a number of images of the temple. Finally, Orissa lost its independence to the Afghans and later to the Mughals. The *maharis*, the temple priests and the servants suffered severe humiliation because there was no security and protection for them any more. Due to lack of social and political stability and lack of royal patronage, the financial status of the *maharis* and their lifestyle deteriorated. They began to lose their spiritual and artistic heritage because, apart from performing, they were forced to lead an immoral lifestyle in the courts of the Mughal rulers for sheer survival.

When the last of the Mughal emperors was defeated and the British took control of the Indian subcontinent, royal patronage of the arts was withdrawn, and performance of dance and music in the temples ceased. The British ruling class who did not understand the art of the *maharis* nor the customs and social environment in which they existed, began to condemn the dance as immoral. Throughout the 19th century, the contrast between Indian and British customs and social practices produced mixed results. By the end of the century, after a campaign led by the British and the Indian social and political reformers, dancing in the temple was banned.

The institution of the *maharis* underwent a period of intense demoralisation and suffered a serious setback, but through the power of the devotion of the *maharis*, the dance was destined to survive.

Left: Shashimoni is the last living mahari.

Above: Late Harapriya was one of the last maharis *of our times.*

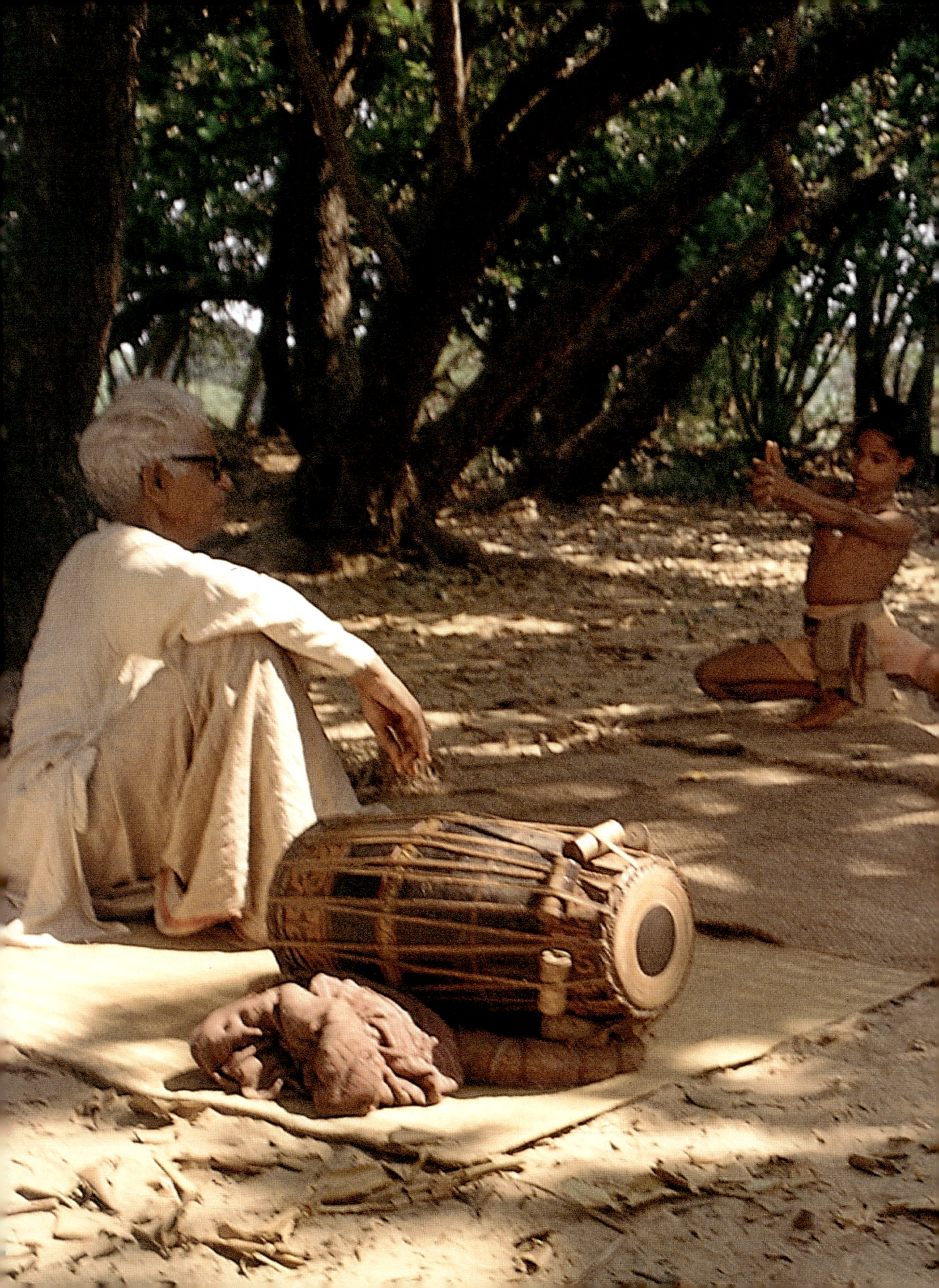

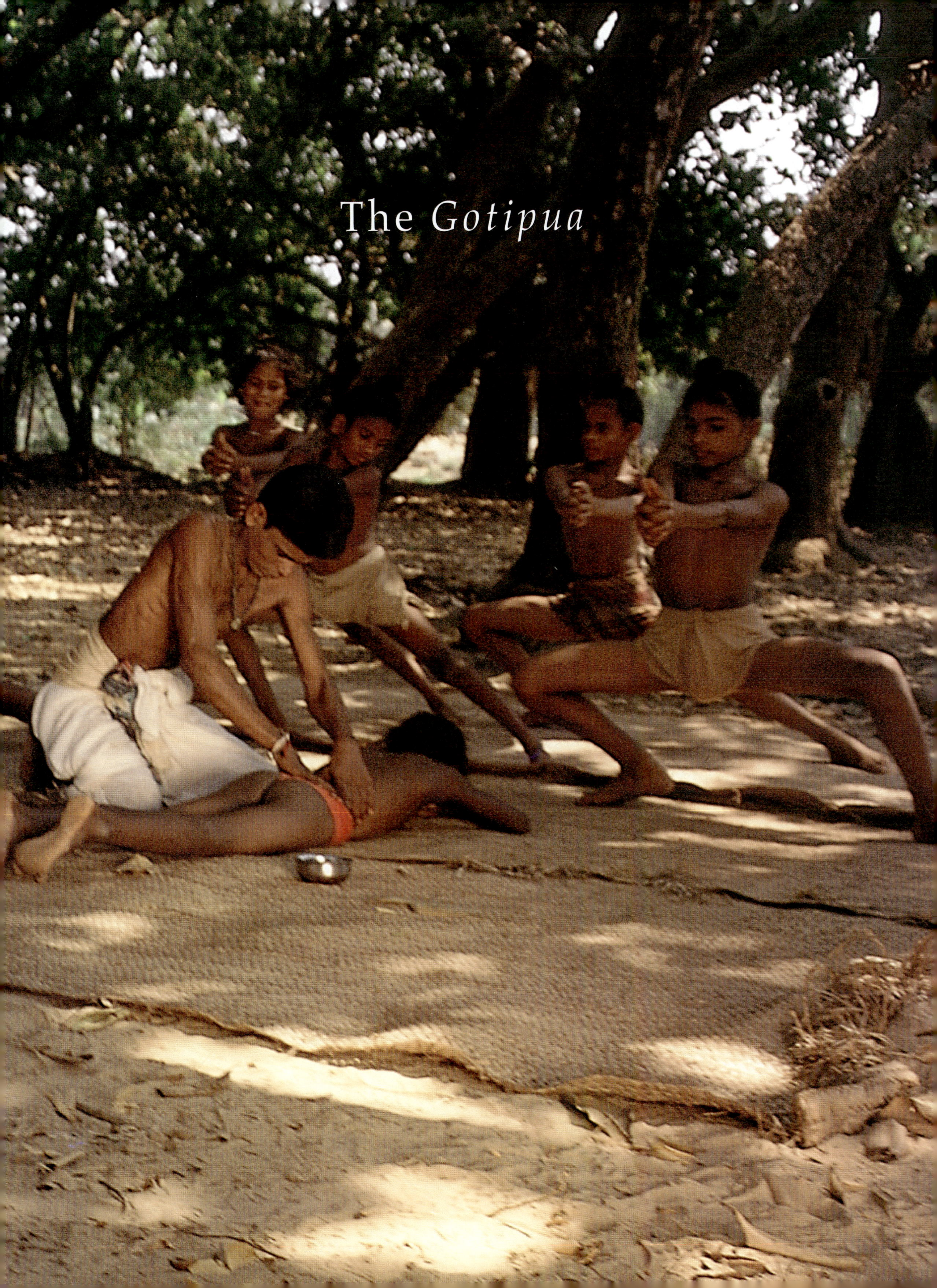

The *Gotipua*

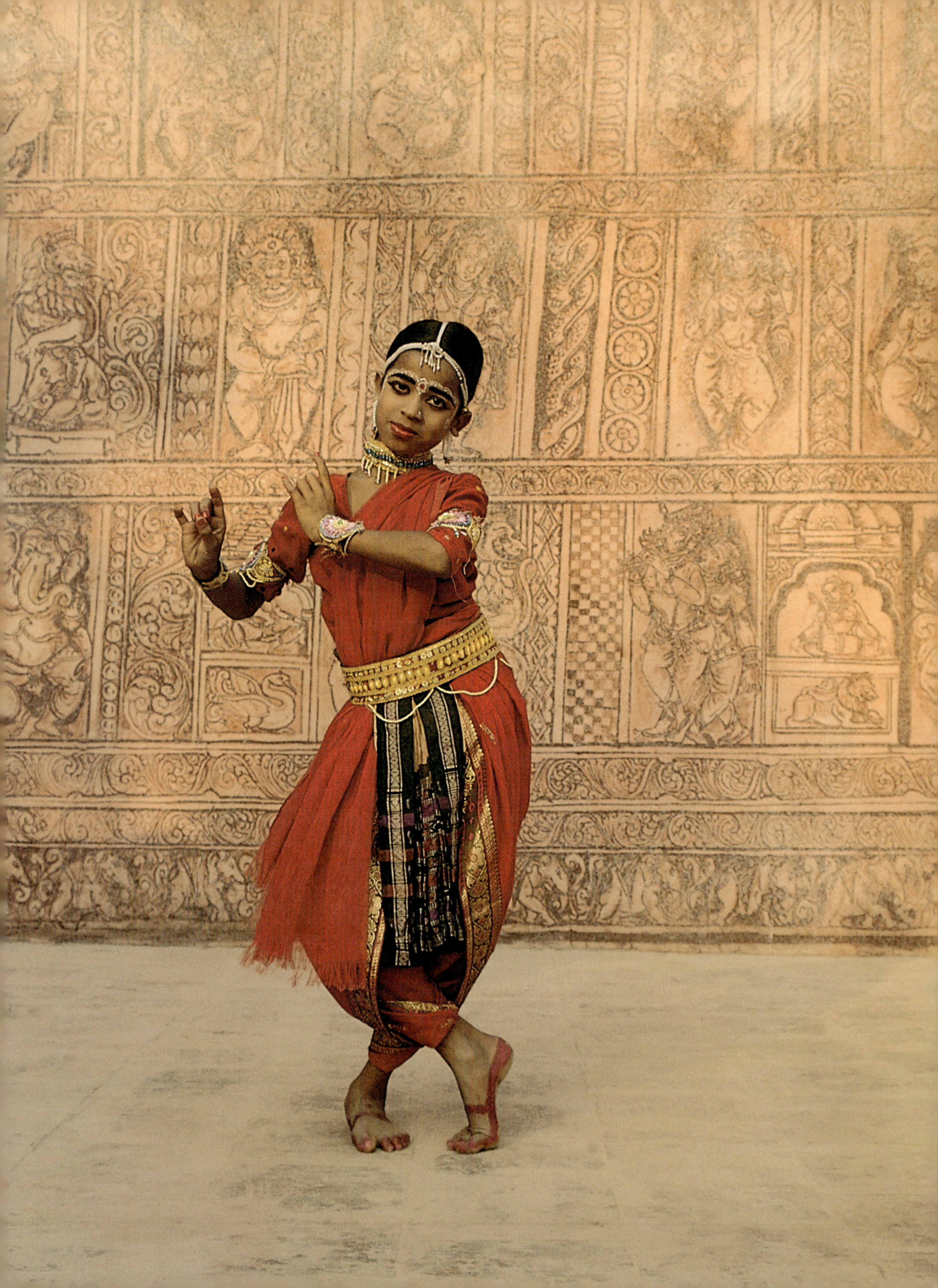

In the history of Odissi dance, there is an unusual and interesting twist that led to the establishment of the *gotipua* dancers as an immensely significant event. Towards the end of the 16th century, the dance of the *gotipuas* gained popularity. The term *goti* means 'single', and *pua* means 'boy'. *Gotipuas,* as such, were young boys, usually between the ages of 6 and 14, who dressed up as girls and were trained in the art of dancing, singing and performing for the general public. They continued to perform till the age of around 16, after which some gave up dancing and others chose to become *gurus* and join theatre troupes.

It is certain that the Odissi dance form as it exists today has its roots in the *gotipua* tradition as much as in the *mahari* tradition. Many of the great Odissi *gurus* of today, were originally trained as *gotipua* dancers.

During the late 15th century, following the various invasions by the Mughals, the rituals and temple traditions were constantly disrupted. It was feared that the purity of the *maharis* would be degraded. Therefore, social pressure was built to create an alternative class of dancers. Hence, the *gotipuas* were created to perform in the festivals and celebrations outside the temple and substitute the *maharis*, as is explained in the following lines:

> For the pleasure of the Yabana kings (i.e., Mughul rulers), male dancers should be sent. Because if the female dancer is touched by such a king, she would lose her religion and would be despised.

Though there are numerous legends and myths about the origin of the *gotipua* dance, it is certain that somehow it was connected with the *mahari* tradition of the Jagannath Temple at Puri. It came into existence during the rule of Ramachandradeva, who is known to have contributed significantly to both *mahari* and *gotipua* traditions. The primary philosophy behind the *gotipua* dance is *sakhi bhava* of the Vaishnav philosophy. *Sakhi bhava* is a concept suggesting that devotion to Lord Krishna is to be expressed in the form of the love of the *gopi* (milkmaid) for the Lord. The devotees consider themselves as the consorts of the Lord. Other theories suggest that because the *maharis* were not allowed to dance outside the temple precincts, the *gotipuas* were needed to fill this gap. The *gotipuas*, however, could not enter the sanctum sanctorum of the temples. Though the *gotipuas* were considered substitutes for the *maharis,* they could not match their dignity and elegance.

The inclusion of the *gotipua* dancers in various festivals associated with the Jagannath Temple became an integral part of the celebrations. During the *Chandan Yatra,* a festival in which Lord Jagannath's idol is taken out on a ceremonial boat ride, the boys would sing, dance and perform on the boat for the deity. Under the patronage of Ramachandradeva, *gotipua* dance grew tremendously—both as an art form and as a part of the local culture of the region.

Preceding double spread: Gotipua *dancers exercising and massaging while Guru Manguni Das watches, in Raghurajpur.*

Left: A gotipua *dancer striking a Krishna pose.*

Following double spread: Gotipua *dancers practising in Raghurajpur.*

Double spread pages 74-75: A gotipua *dancer in the process of preparing for a performance.*

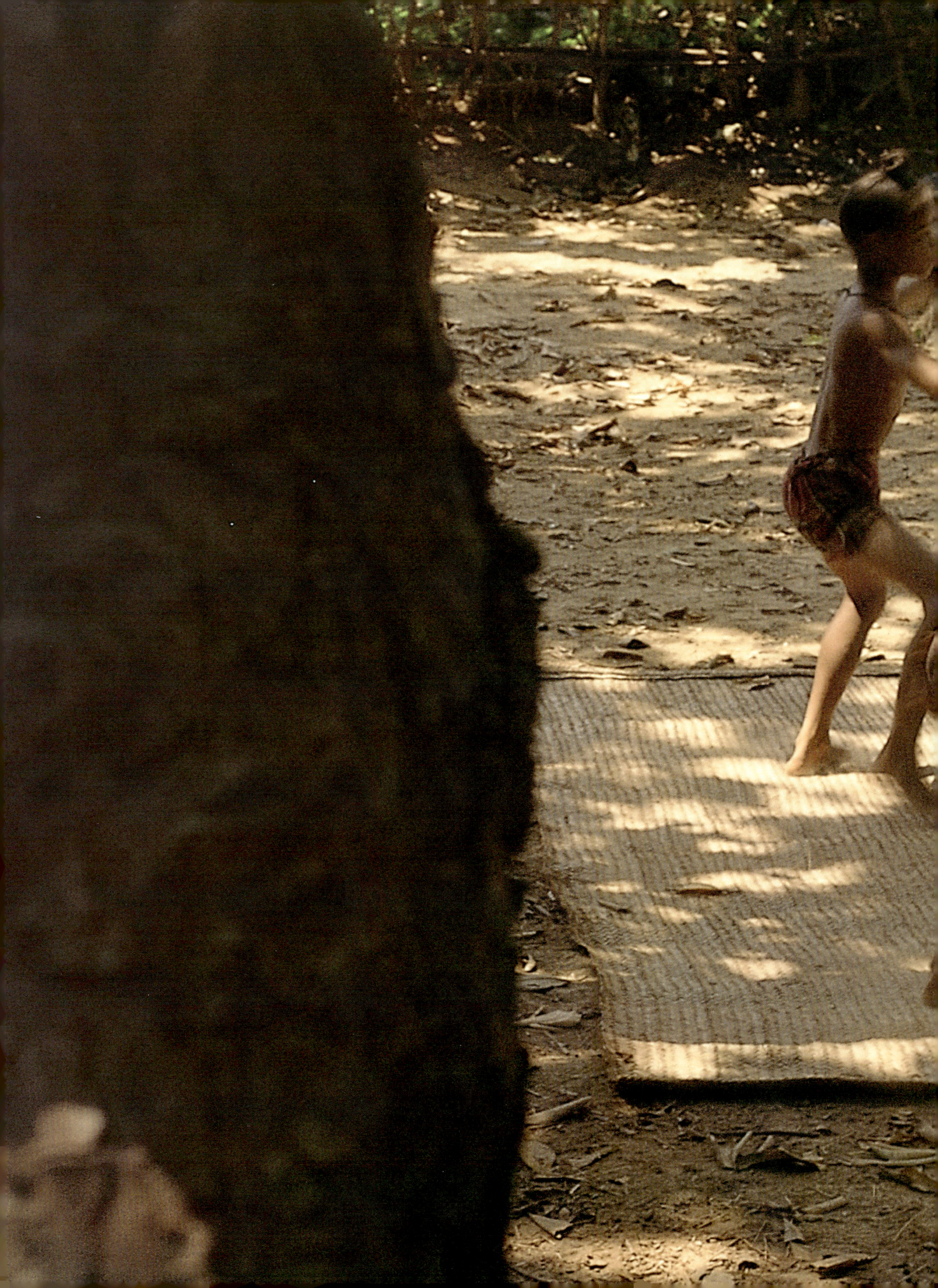

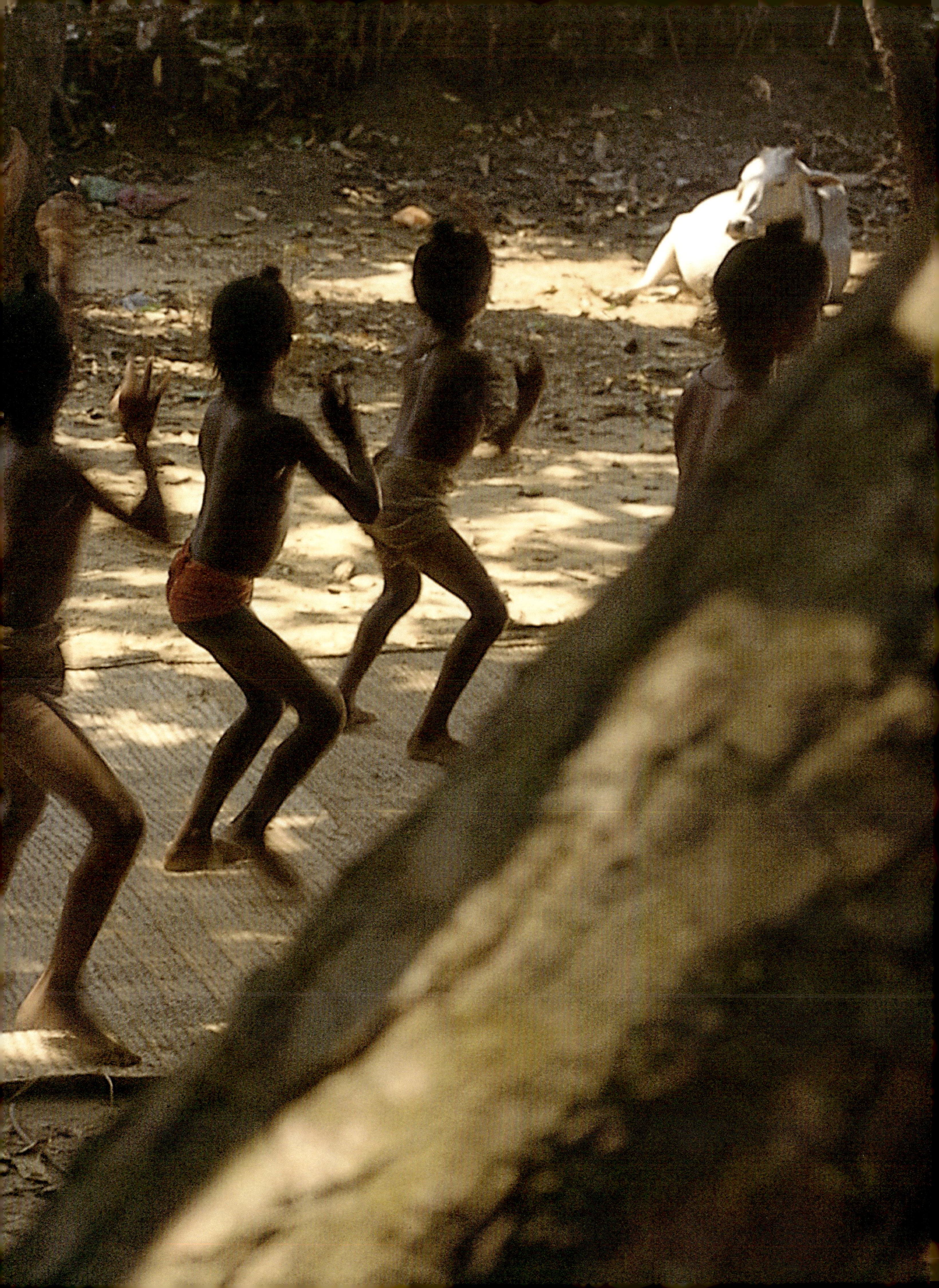

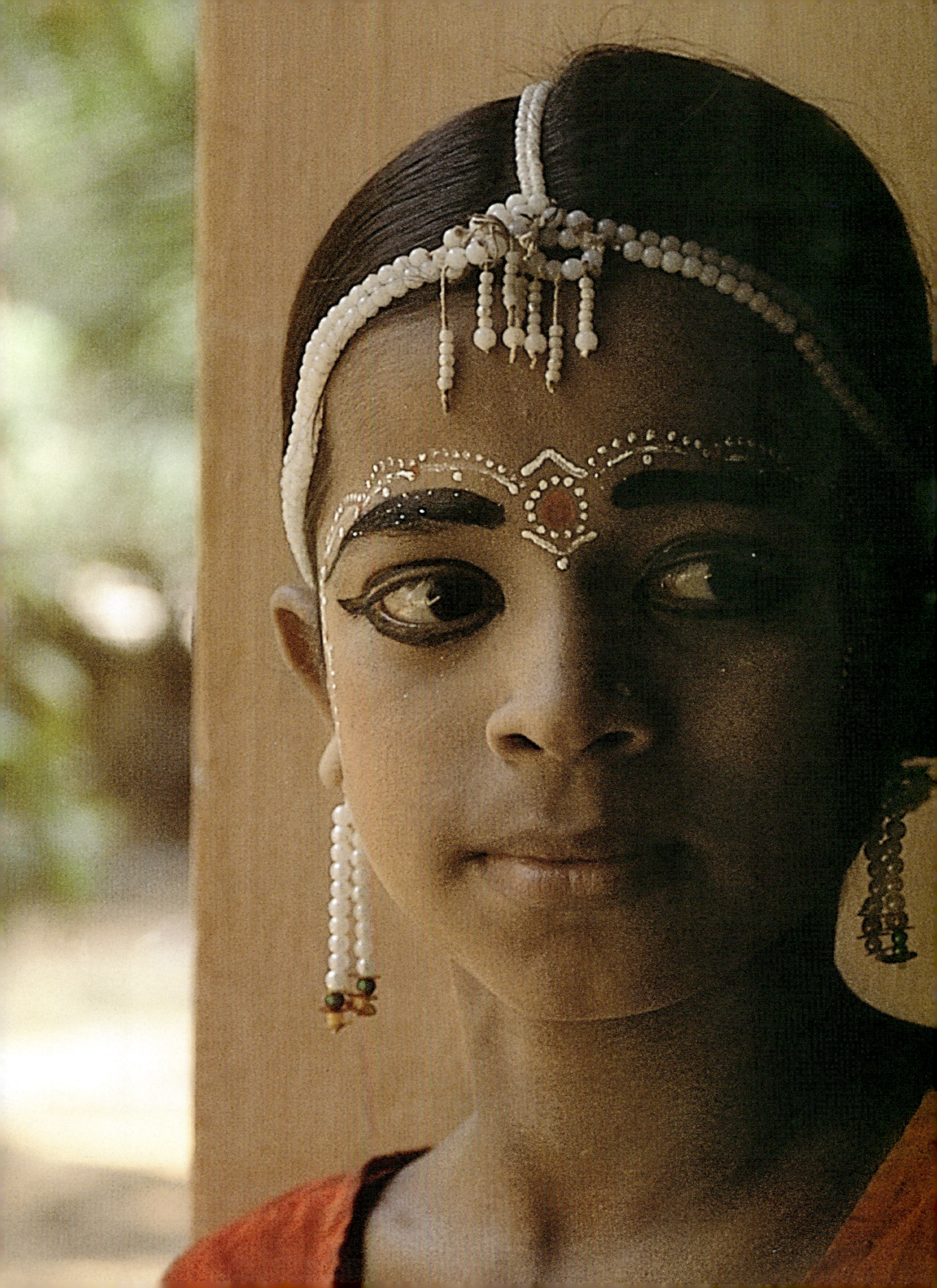

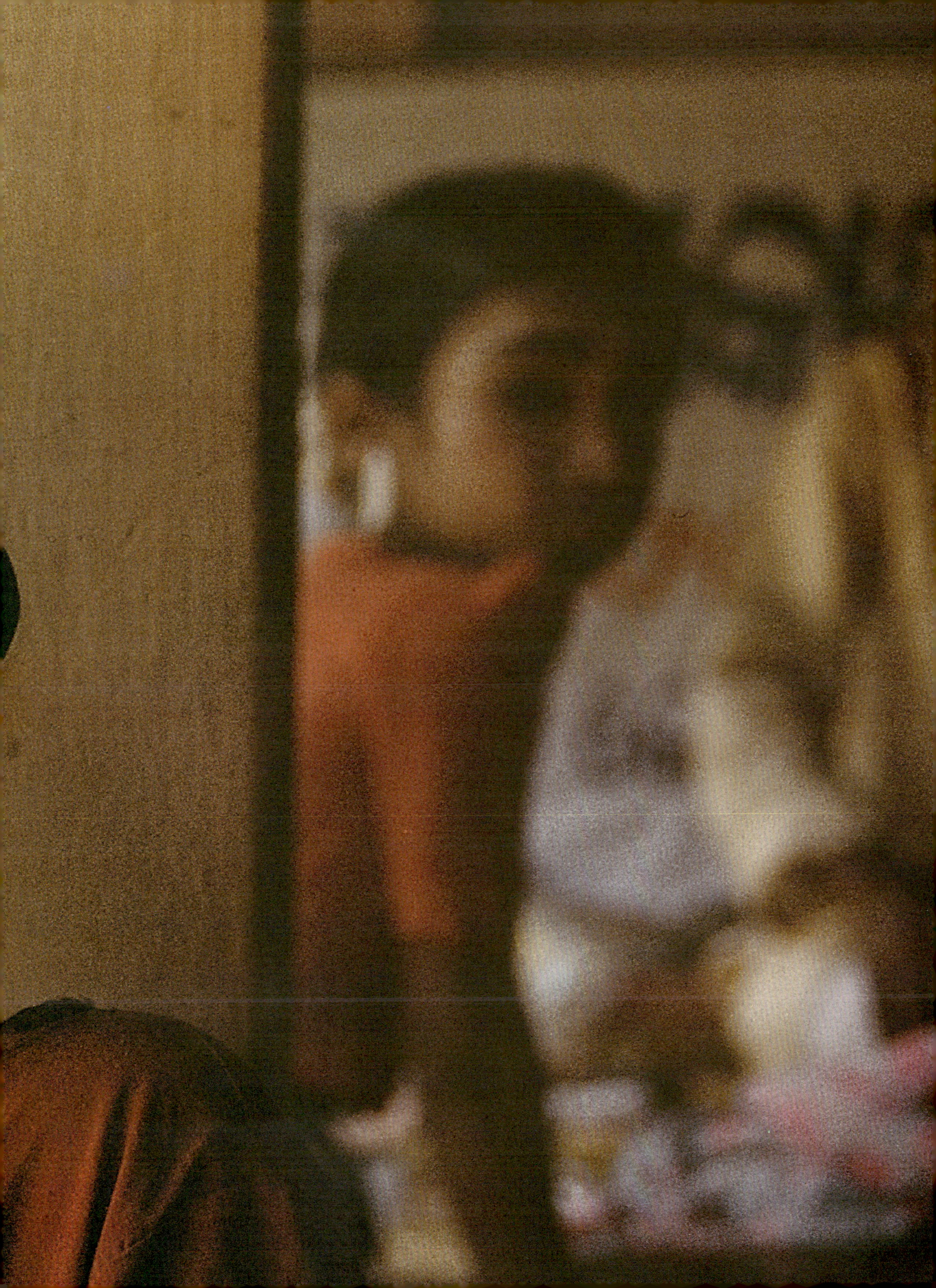

Gotipua troupes travelled all over Orissa popularising the dance form. They sang songs written by eminent Oriya poets like Gopal Krishna Patnaik, Banamali Das and Kavisurya Baladeva Ratha popularising Vaishnav philosophy.

Ramachandradeva is also credited with the construction of numerous *akhadas*, institutions similar to gymnasiums or clubs, for the training of *gotipuas*. The *akhadas* became not only a key factor in the evolution of the *gotipua* dance but also became great centres of cultural activities.

The influence of *akhadas* on the dancing of *gotipuas* can be seen in the *bandha nritya*, meaning 'dance with difficult movements'. *Bandha nritya* involves acrobatic poses and movements. *Abhinaya Chandrika* and *Natya Shastra* make references to various positions called *karanas* that are frequently seen in the *bandha nritya* of the *gotipua* repertoire. Besides the encouragement from the *akhadas* and religious *maths* (monastries), the *zamindars* or the landed gentry also patronised them and maintained *gotipua* troupes.

During the 19th century, the dance of the *gotipuas* came under the influence of the *sakhi nach* of southern Orissa, which was already in a state of decadence under the influence of the *devadasis* of the Telugu region. These influences

Lending a helping hand to a co-dancer before a gotipua *performance.*

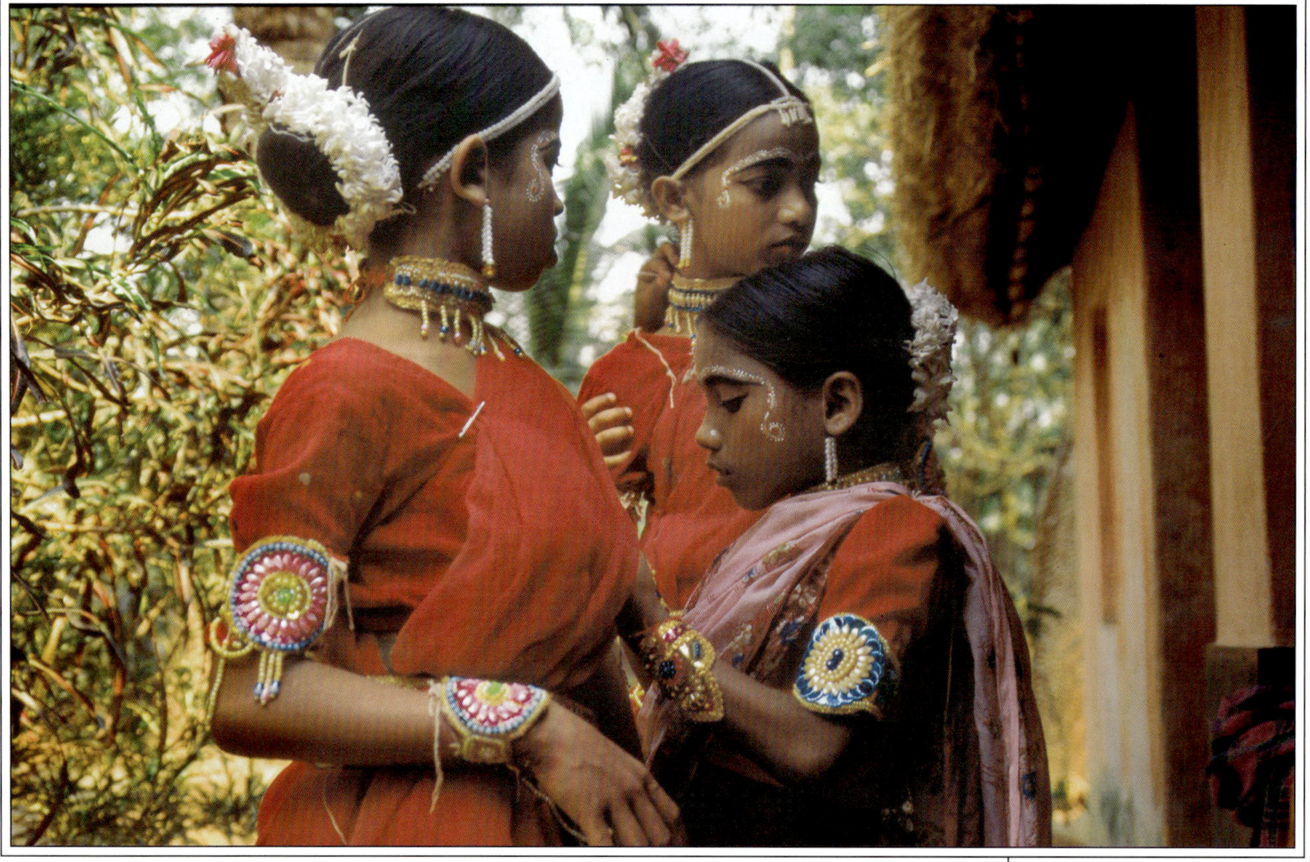

corrupted the *gotipua* dance during the closing years of the last century, even as popular cinema added insult to injury.

However, the *gotipua* dance has managed to survive as a style in its own right and continues to play an important part in the cultural life of Orissa even today. The present-day Odissi *gurus* were at one time *gotipua* dancers and because of their continued involvement, including the performances in *raslila* parties, the art of Odissi survived and metamorphosed into the present-day form of Odissi dance.

Below and following double spread: Gotipua *dancers performing the* bandha nritya.

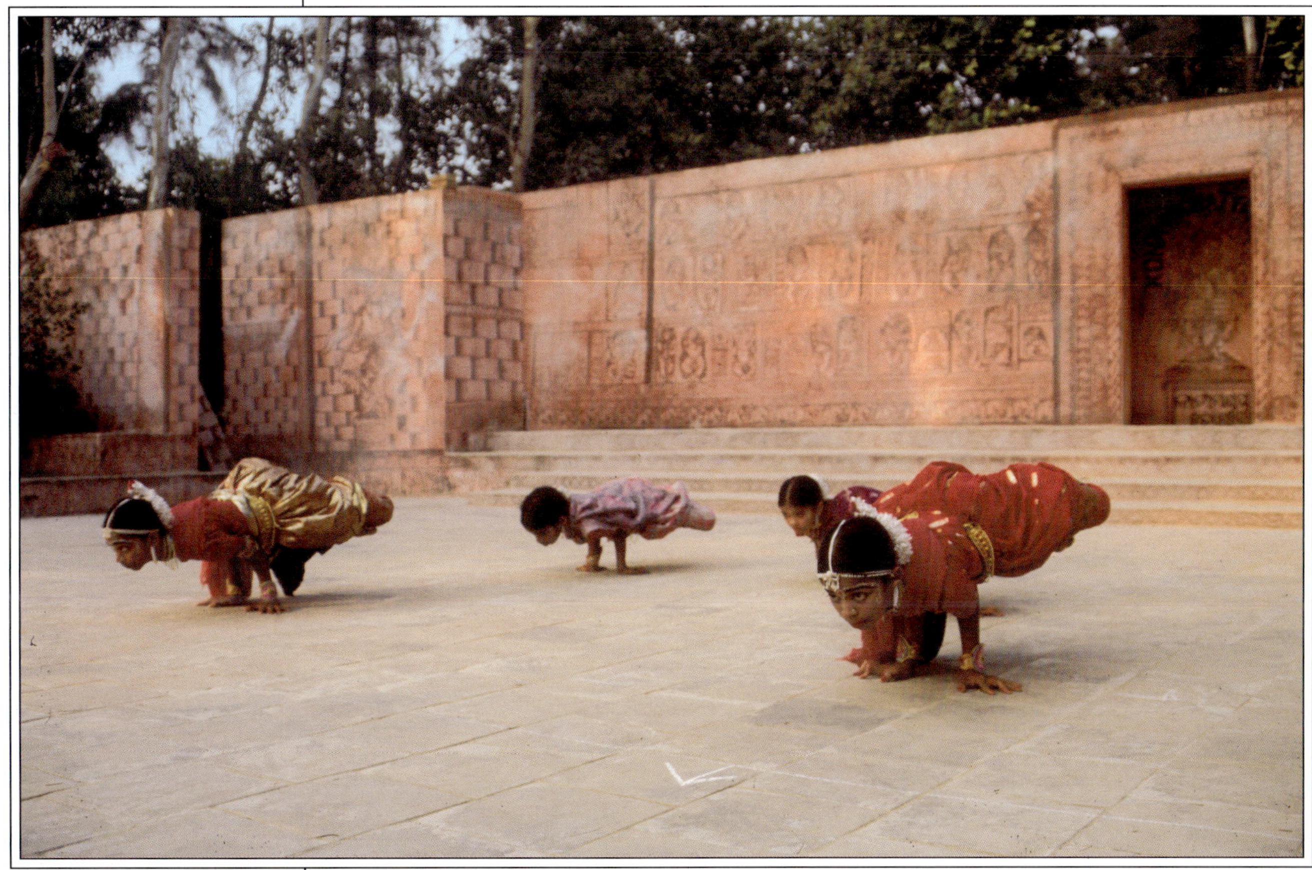

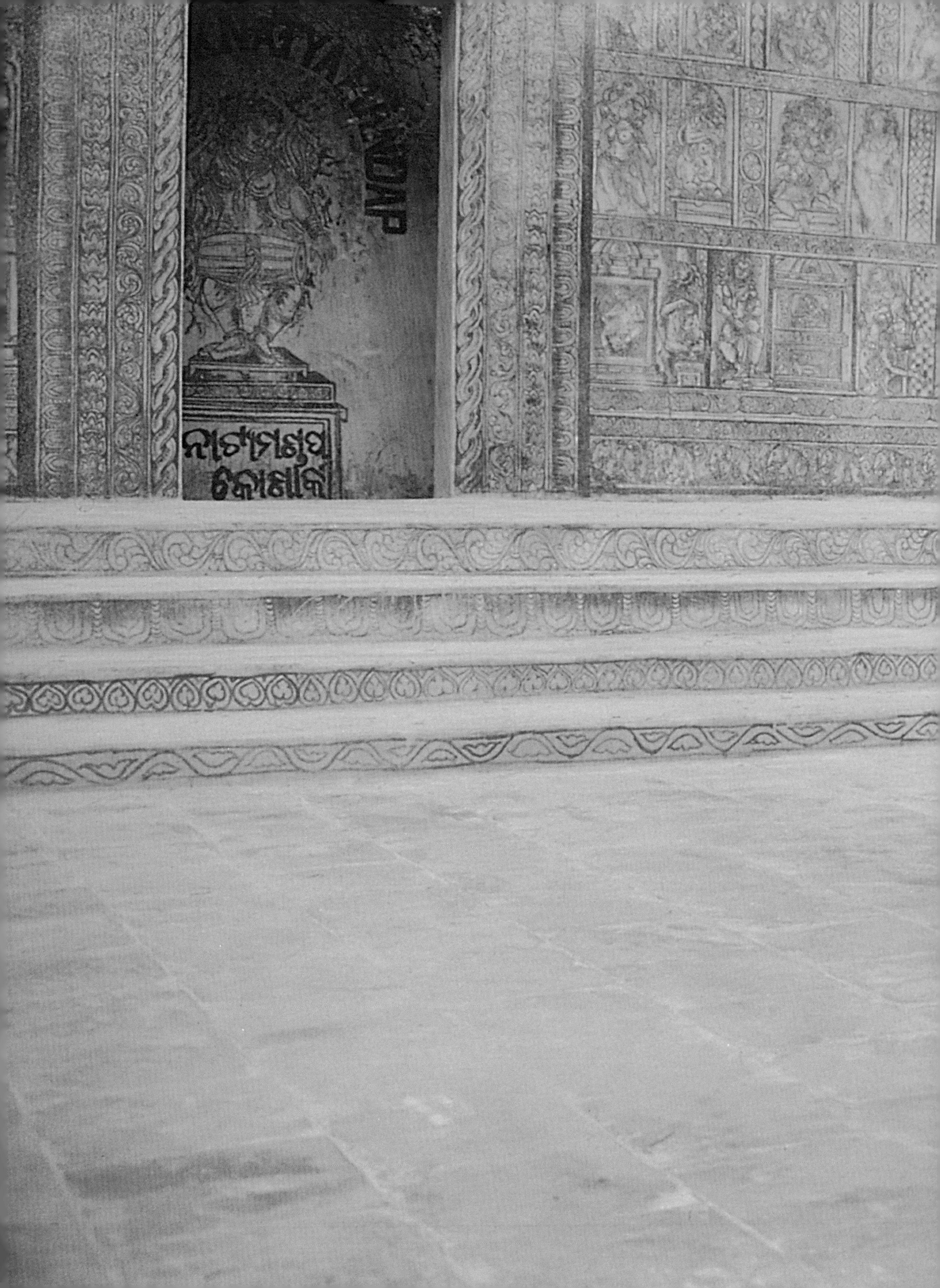
ନାଟମଣ୍ଡପ
କୋଣାର୍କ

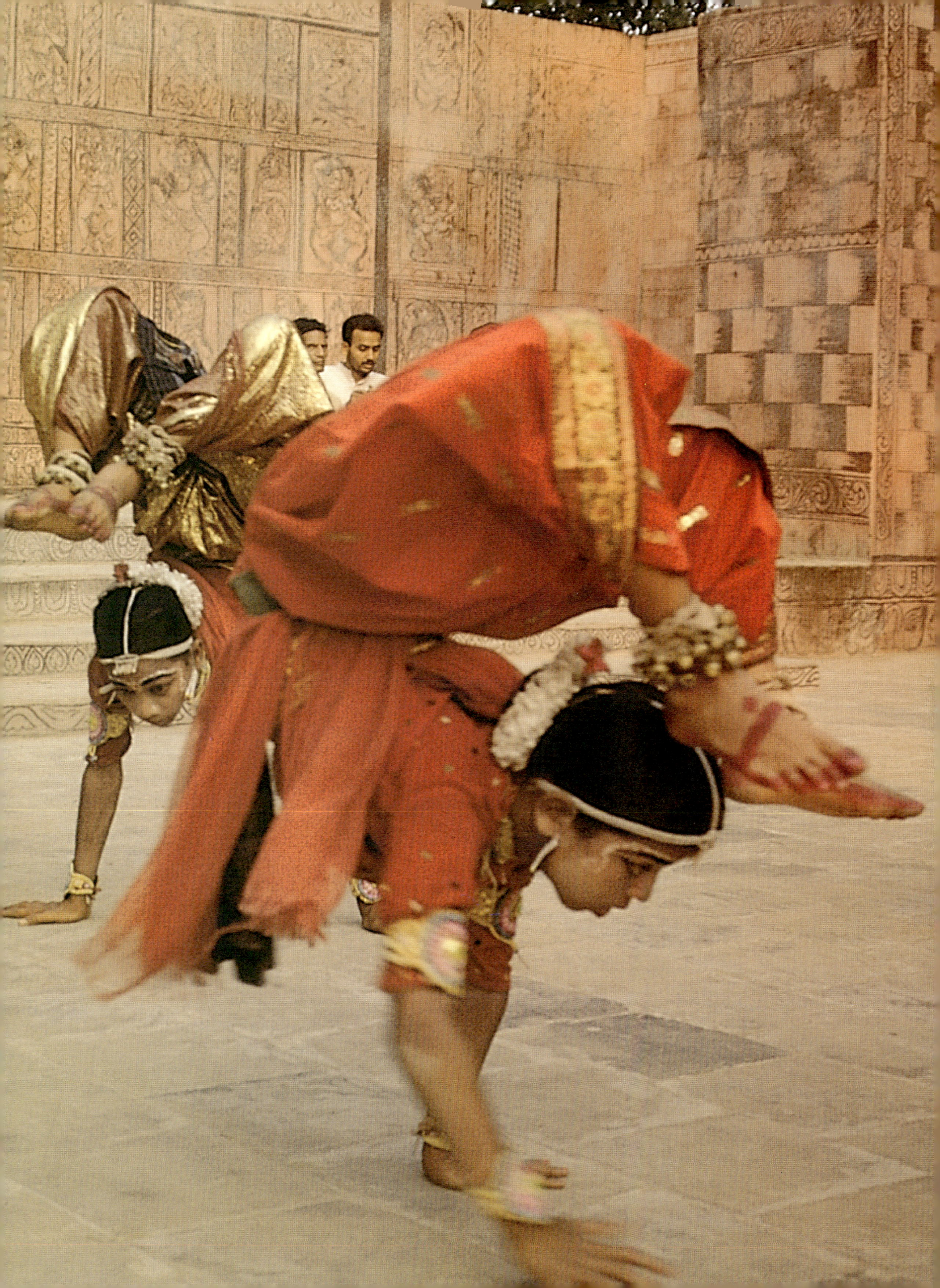

THE DECLINE OF ODISSI

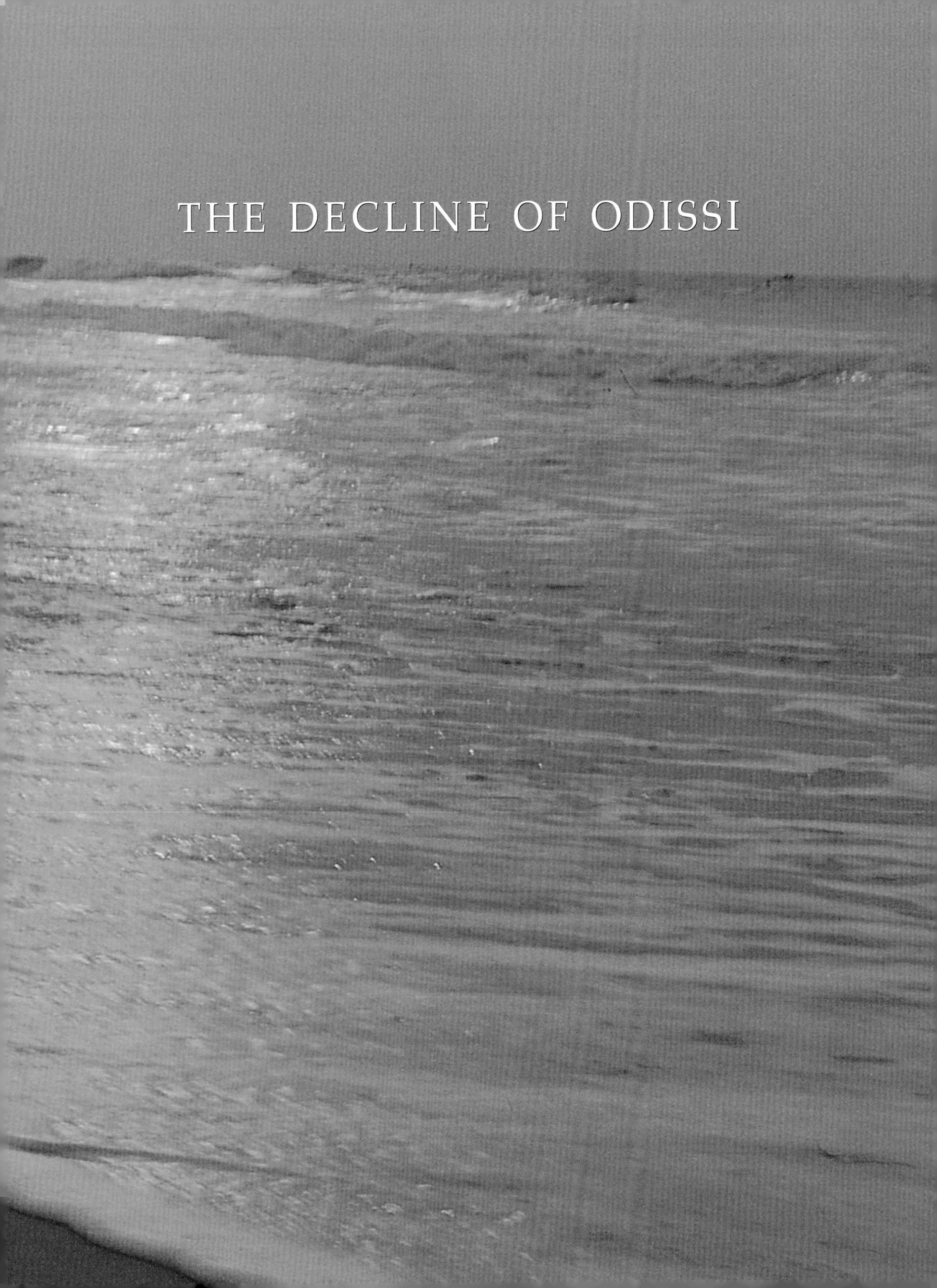

With the decline of the Gajapati kings in the early 16th century, the Mughal rule made its way into Orissa, establishing the beginning of a Hindu-Muslim struggle for power that would result in alternating waves of destruction and revival of the Jagannath Temple and all the traditions associated with it. Because of their artistry, skill and education, *maharis* were respected and admired but also sought after by the princes, courtiers and scholars who would come to invade the Indian subcontinent in the following years.

In 1568, Orissa lost its independence to the Afghans and experienced the destruction of hundreds of Hindu shrines. The deities in the Jagannath Temple at Puri were burnt and cast into the sea, the temple defaced and destroyed, and the temple servants humiliated. The services of the temple were suspended for several years.

Beautifully carved sculptures in Hindu temples suffered great damage during the Mughal invasion of Orissa.

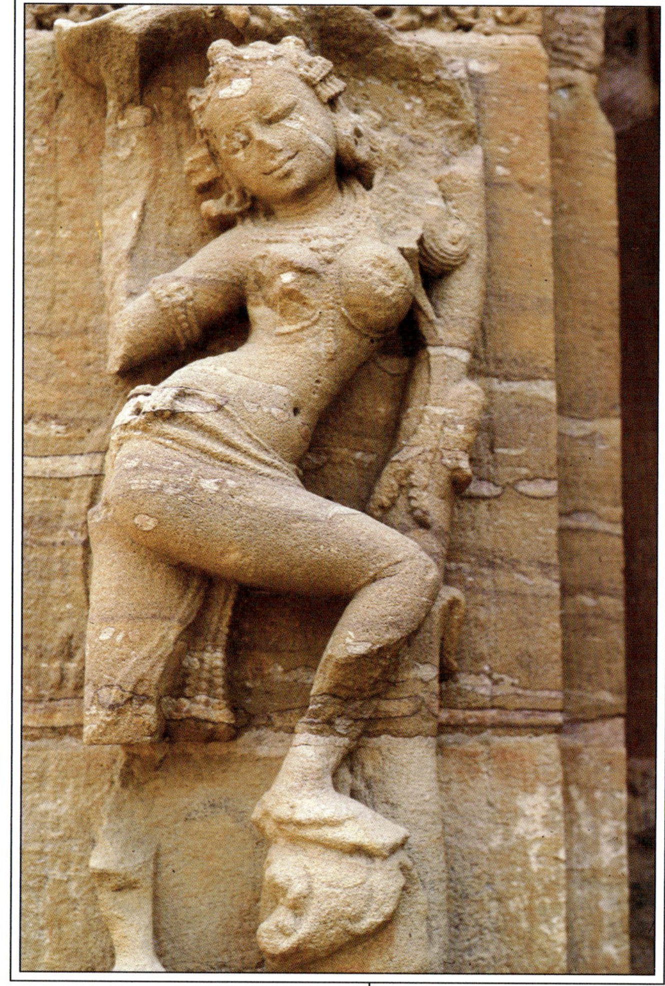

Though the *mahari* tradition temporarily regained patronage and was revived under the rule of Ramachandradeva and later by staunch Hindu Marathas, the recurring struggle with the Mughal invaders of Orissa considerably weakened the stability and spiritual purity of the tradition.

During the Mughal rule , the reputation of the temple dancers fell into disrepute, and the dance was commonly accepted as 'an amusement, an entertainment' at its best, and an instrument of indiscipline, temptation and vice, at its worst. The British ruling class, who neither understood the art of the *maharis*, nor the customs and social environment in which they existed, began to condemn the dance as immoral.

Madala Panji, the records of the Jagannath Temple, refer to the atrocities perpetrated by the Mughal invaders, and historians like Abdul Fazl have left accounts of the mayhem. Though for some time, the Bhoi king, Ramachandradeva, was in power and had once again installed the idols in the temple, after his rule, great political turmoil prevailed for the next 300 years, when the Mughals, the Marathas and the British ruled over Orissa. The British took over Orissa from the Marathas in 1830. However, they didn't interfere with the temple service (L.S.S.O. Malley ICS, *Bengal District Gazetteer*, Puri, pp. 102–104).

It was when the last of the Mughal emperor was defeated and the British took full control of the Indian subcontinent that royal patronage to the arts was withdrawn and ritual dance and music in the temples curtailed.

Throughout the 19th century, the contrast between Indian and British customs and social practices produced mixed results. The British encouraged Indian families of wealth and status to provide their young women the opportunity for education, but 'it was not considered seemly for ordinary women to learn to read, sing or dance.' Interestingly, one of the great objections against the education of respectable Indian girls was that they might be mistaken for dancing girls, who alone could read, write, sing and play a musical instrument.

By the end of the century, the concerns of morality-conscious Hindus combined with the zeal of Christian missionaries, who could not imagine that faith could be expressed through so 'immodest and voluptuous a medium as dance', led to the virtual demise of the *maharis*. In 1878, William Ward Hunter wrote: 'In the pillared hall, dancing girls enliven the idol's repast. With their airy gyrations and their rolling eyes, they put the modest female worshipper to shame.'

It is true that many prostitutes, some loosely connected to the *mahari* community, had begun 'nautch dancing'—a commercial version of dance—to lure customers. But the leaders of what was to be the anti-nautch movement hardly made distinctions between one form of the dance and another. One campaign led by the British and Indian social and political reformers went so far as to ban temple dancing in certain regions.

The art of dance and music suffered on account of political instability—the Muslim invasion, desecration of the temples, loss of independence and lack of patronage to dancers. Consequently, the quality of dance deteriorated and by the time the Odissi dance came to be known to the outside world, it was a mere shadow of its glorious past.

A priest at the Jagannath Temple in Puri remarked:

'*Mahari* dance was not an ordinary dance. It was a dance of substance. The hand movements and dramatic gestures were a part of our worship. It is no longer that.'

And *mahari* Hari Priya solemnly commented:

'Our hearts are saddened but what can we do? Just a single person cannot sustain the tradition. If so, I would have done it already.'

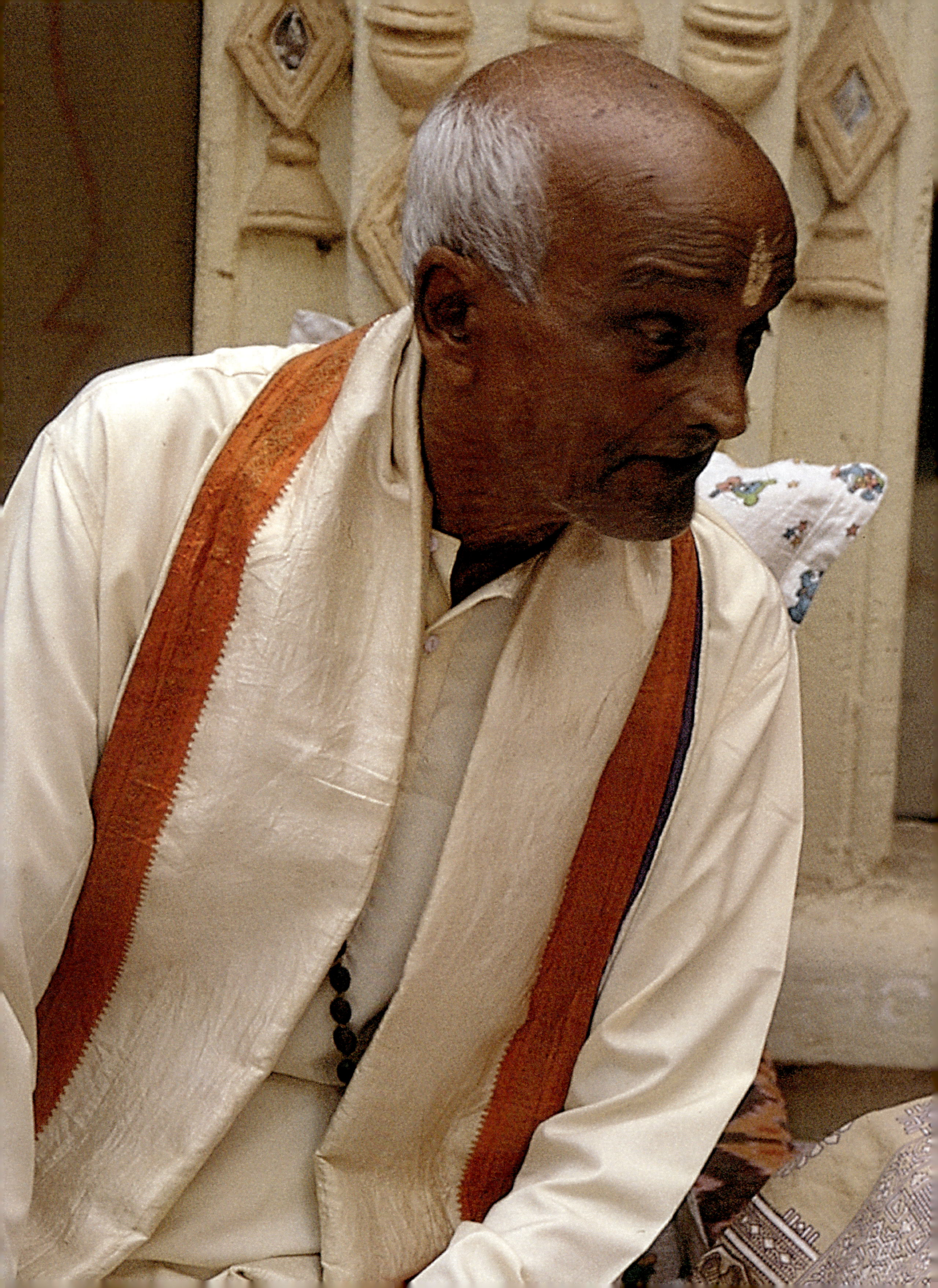

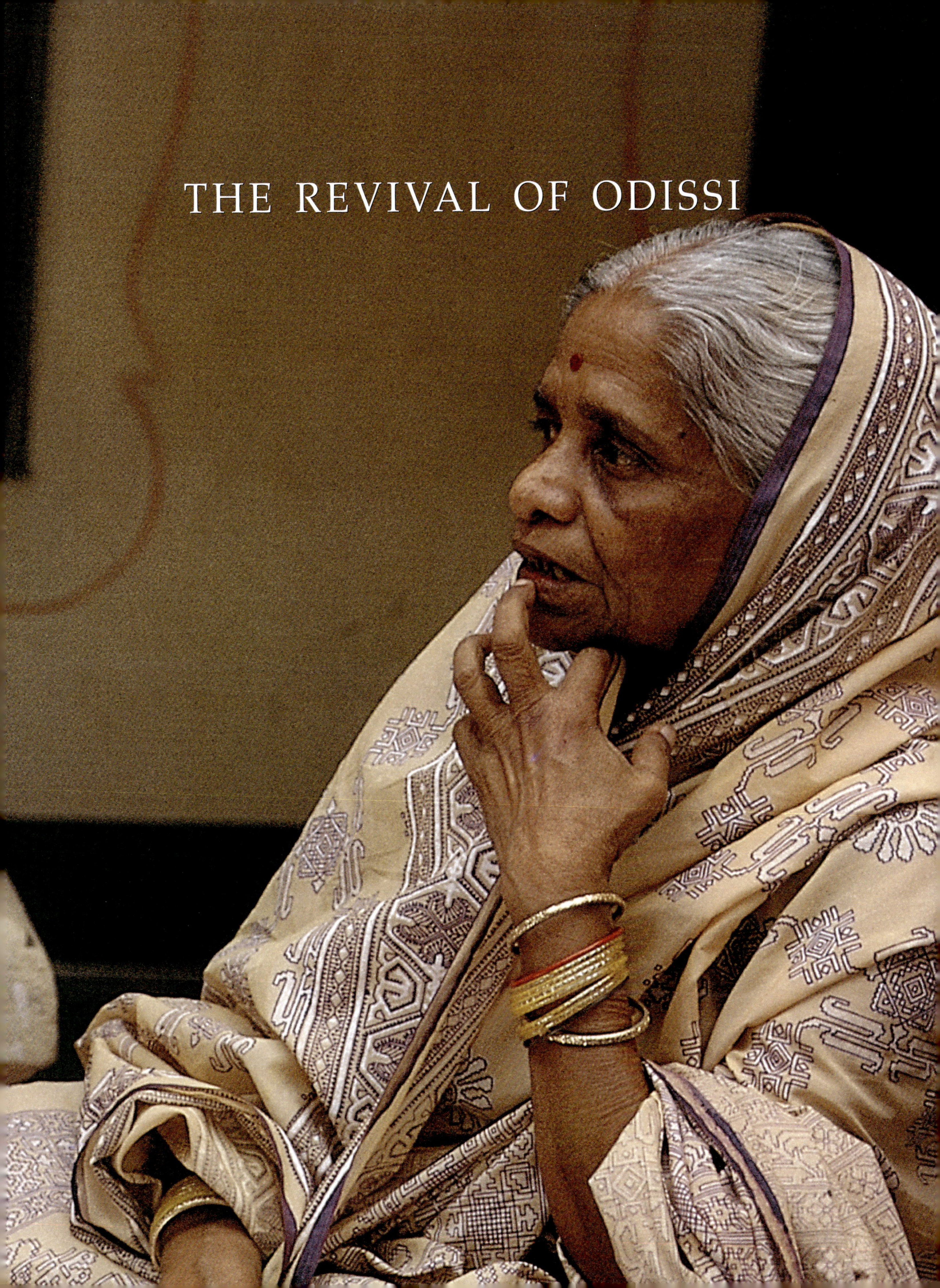

THE REVIVAL OF ODISSI

The year of India's Independence, 1947, saw the people of the new nation increasingly interested in rebuilding a cultural heritage that had diminished under centuries of foreign domination. The independence movement had sparked a renewed pride in all things indigenous, and poetry, literature, music and dance were celebrated as the survivors of a rich cultural tradition that began to evolve over 2000 years ago. The indigenous classical Indian dances became a top concern of the cultural revival.

The dance form of Odissi is the product of a motivated effort by *gurus*, leading artists, scholars and concerned patrons. Although the tradition of dance and music in Orissa had fallen into grave disrepute during the British period, the authentic lineage of the classical legacy was preserved by certain distinguished *gurus* and artist families who had continued to practise the art. *Gurus* such as late Pankaj Charan Das, late Kelucharan Mohapatra, late Deba Prasad Das and Mayadhar Raut, and dancers such as late Indrani Rehman, late Sanjukta Panigrahi, Priyambada Mohanty, Sonal Mansingh and Kumkum Das *née* Mohanty spearheaded the movement that eventually brought Odissi into the limelight once again.

Since the late 1950s, through the efforts of these *gurus*, along with a host of scholars that included the Hungarian Indologist and dance critic Dr Charles Fabri, scholar and poet Kavichandra Kalicharan Patnaik, poet and historian Mayadhar Mansingh and scholar / dancer Dhirendra Nath Patnaik, Odissi eventually came to be known as one of the hidden jewels of India's cultural legacy. In 1954, when Dr Charles Fabri described Odissi as 'one of the most perfect surviving Indian classical dances', he inspired a whole generation of talented dancers who would bring Odissi dance to the forefront of the national artistic consciousness.

The *mahari* and *gotipua* forms gradually converged as dancers and *gurus* became influenced by, and started learning from, both the styles, and out of this blending emerged the present Odissi form. Late Guru Pankaj Charan Das, who was the *guru* of *gurus*, was a great example of the synthesis of two traditions. Even though he was a not a trained *gotipua* dancer but the adopted son of a *mahari*, he made dance history by merging the two traditions in the present-day Odissi.

Among the first batch of girls to be trained in the dances of Orissa was Priyambada Mohanty whose accomplishments were of critical importance to the evolution of the Odissi dance form. In 1954 at the Inter-University Youth Festival in New Delhi, young Priyambada Mohanty, accompanied by her *guru*, Deba Prasad Das, gave a performance that would instantly propel Odissi to

Preceding double spread: Guru of Gurus, Shree Pankaj Charan Das with his wife.

Above: Charles Fabri rediscovered the Odissi dance.

the national dance scene. It caught the attention of some very important scholars and critics. Dr Charles Fabri, praised the unknown dance form as 'strikingly original'.

That was the beginning of a long running debate on the authenticity and validity of Odissi as a classical dance. Over the next several years, *gurus*, scholars, patrons and lovers of dance, who were increasing in number, came together for the cause of Odissi under the banner *Jayantika*. *Jayantika* was a vibrant movement that sought to vitalise the Odissi dance form and fight for its recognition. Braving the opposition of a number of conservatives who had condemned the dance as a 'cheap imitation' of the other classical styles, *Jayantika* worked hard for many years to re-establish and rectify the technique, strengthen the structure, the repertoire, costumes and ornamentation of the Odissi style along classical lines. Late Kavichandra Kalicharan Patnaik, a distinguished Oriya poet, playwright and musicologist who was leading this movement, delved into research on the ancient dance *shastras*, or texts, and found evidence corroborating Odissi's classical status. He also discovered more detailed guidelines as to how the dance form needed to be restructured. According to Dhirendra Nath Patnaik, Kavichandra Kalicharan Patnaik coined the name Odissi—meaning that which is peculiar to Orissa. Guru Kelucharan Mohapatra with his inimitable sense of rhythm and gift for playing the *pakhawaj*, Guru Deba Prasad Das with his lyrical and graceful style of movement, and Guru Mayadhar Raut with his unparalleled expressional choreographies, and scholars like D.N. Patnaik were all extremely active in *Jayantika*. It was from the hands of these exceptional *gurus* and scholars that the Odissi repertoire and technique emerged. Although Guru Pankaj Charan Das did not interact with the *Jayantika* group on a regular basis, his style and graceful movements were indirectly incorporated into the new Odissi as all the *gurus* who worked for *Jayantika* were at one time or another his trainees.

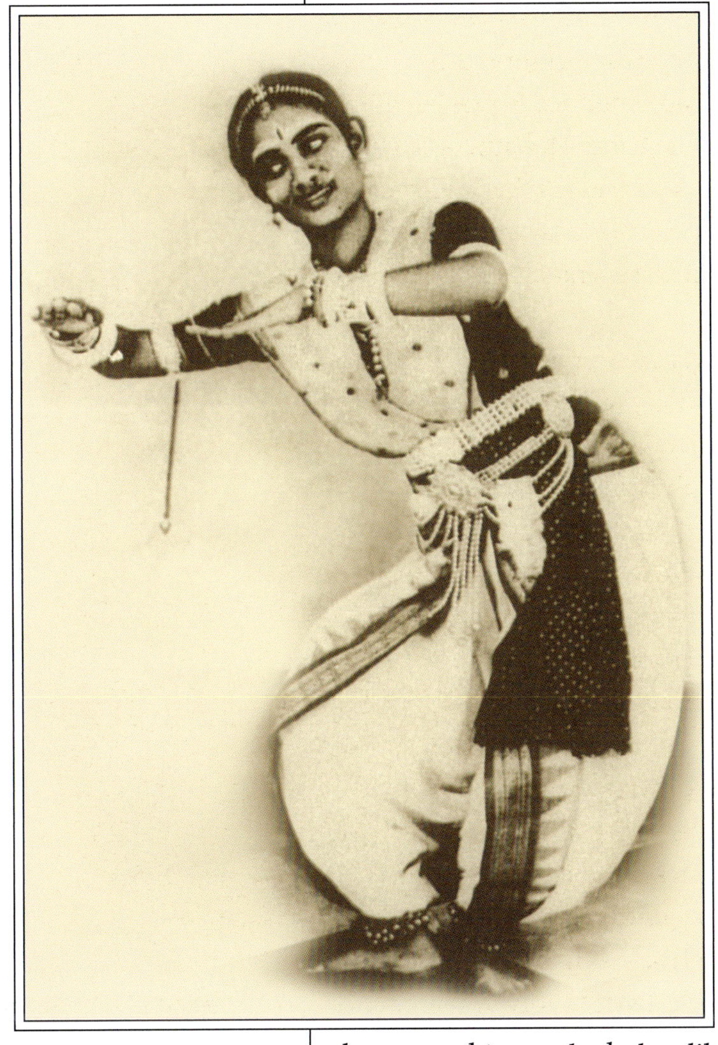

Above: Priyambada Mohanty represented the Odissi dance at the Delhi University dance competition held in the early 1950s for the first time.
Photo courtesy: Priyambada Mohanty

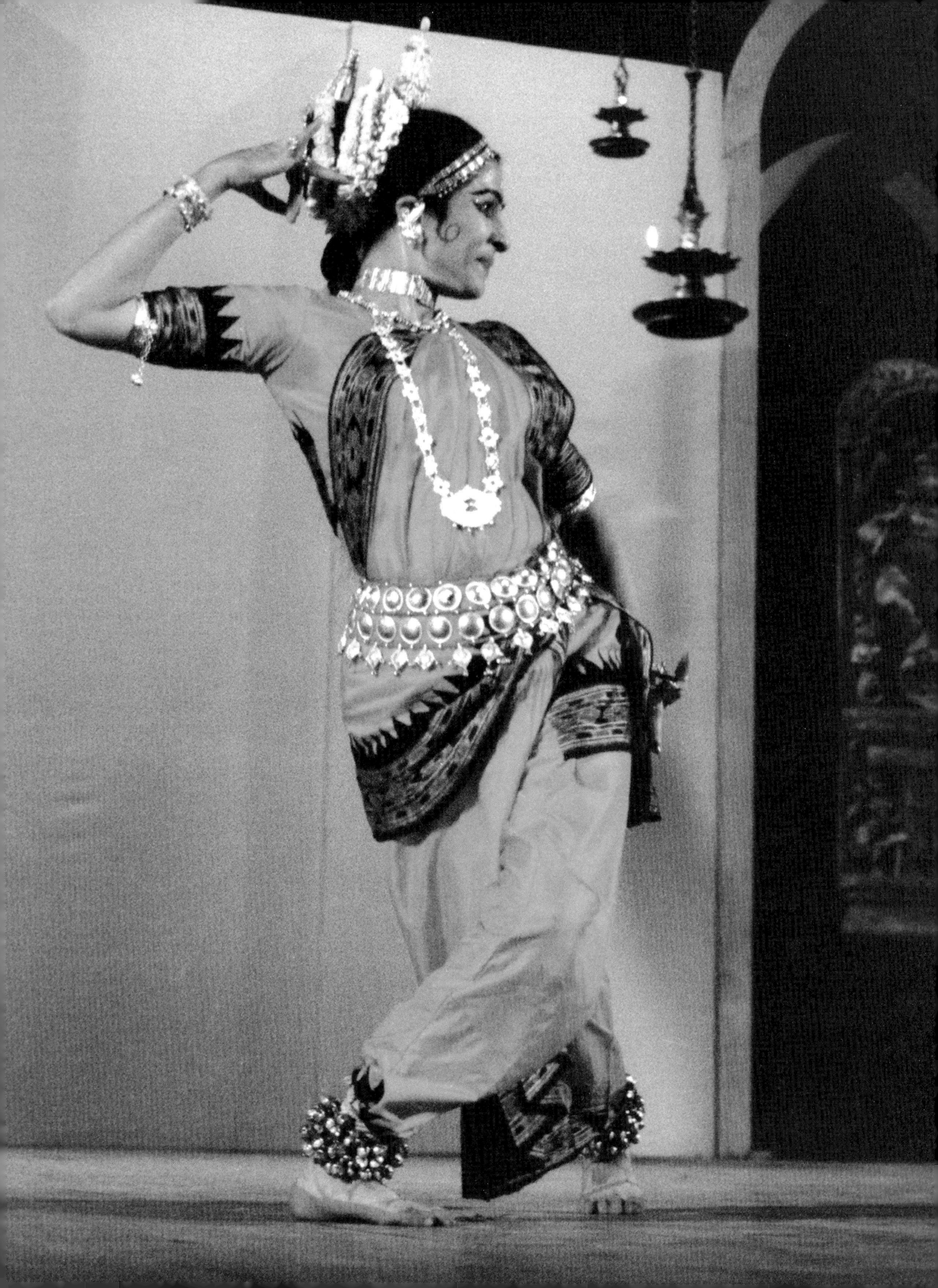

During the next two decades, the technique and repertoire of Odissi were fully reconstructed and the art was not only accepted as a classical style, but also hailed as one of the nation's most lyrical, graceful and stirring dance forms.

Concerns among contemporary scholars on dance cite arguments about 'the modern myth of ancient heritage' of not just Odissi, but all the classical dance forms of India. The main concern among these historians is the popularly accepted belief of the antiquity of the classical art forms. But perhaps the very beauty of Odissi as a classical dance form is because its existence is the product of 'contemporary interpretations and interpolations based on restricted repertoires and knowledge of temple dancer, i.e., the *mahari*, and its extensions of the expertise of *gotipuas*'. The technique of Odissi has been consolidated, and the debate about its classical status has faded. The reconstruction of Odissi, like the other classical dance forms, in no way diminishes the vast achievements of the scholars, *gurus*, and dancers of the art, but instead establishes a remarkable synthesis of the contemporary with the ancient, of tradition with modernity.

Those who have been fortunate enough to see the performance of Guru Kelucharan Mohapatra or seen Guru Pankaj Charan Das singing and practising his *abhinaya* would be able to understand that the depth and beauty of Odissi, despite the fact that it has gone through so much upheaval, lies in its spirituality and intense devotion. And that makes the very essence of what Odissi is today.

Left: Sanjukta Panigrahi in an imposing Odissi posture.
Photo courtesy: Sangeet Natak Akademi, New Delhi

Below: Guru Kelucharan Mohapatra playing the mardala.

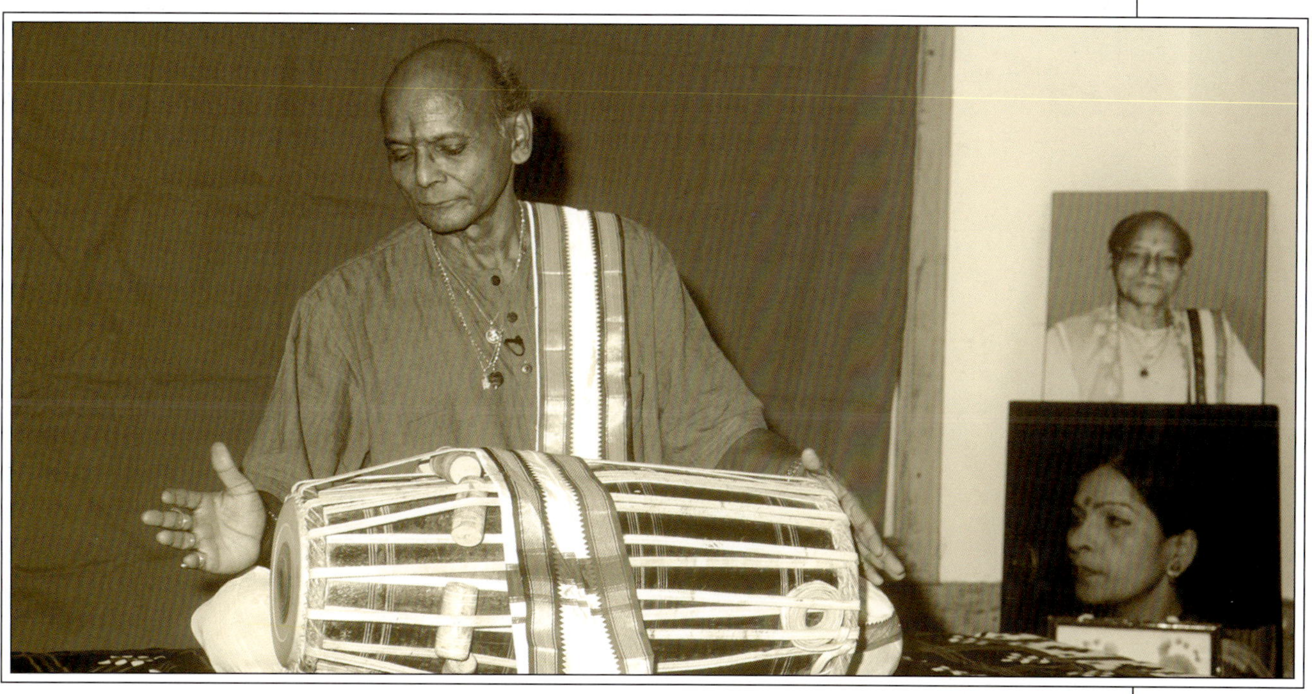

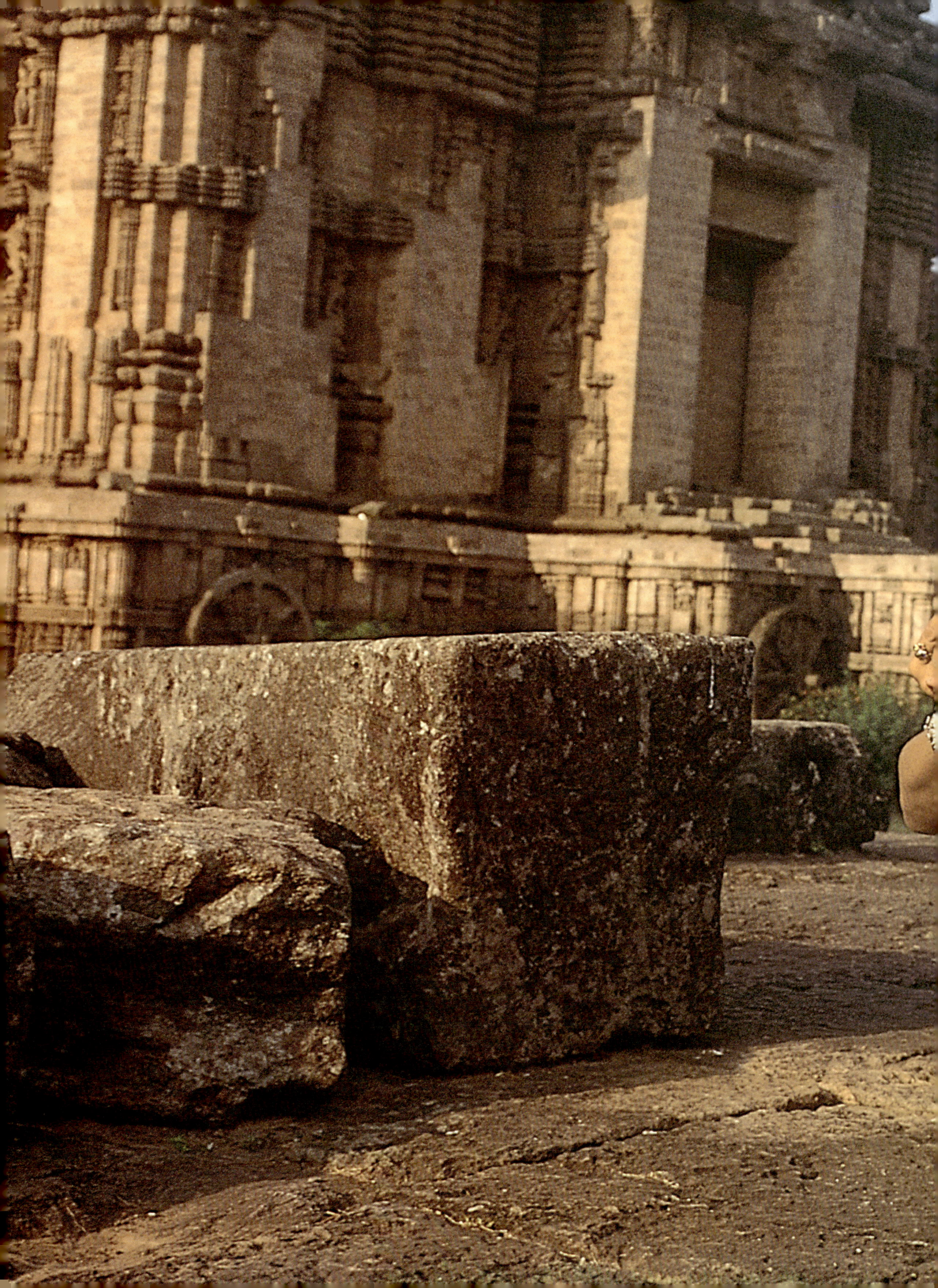

AESTHETICS OF ODISSI

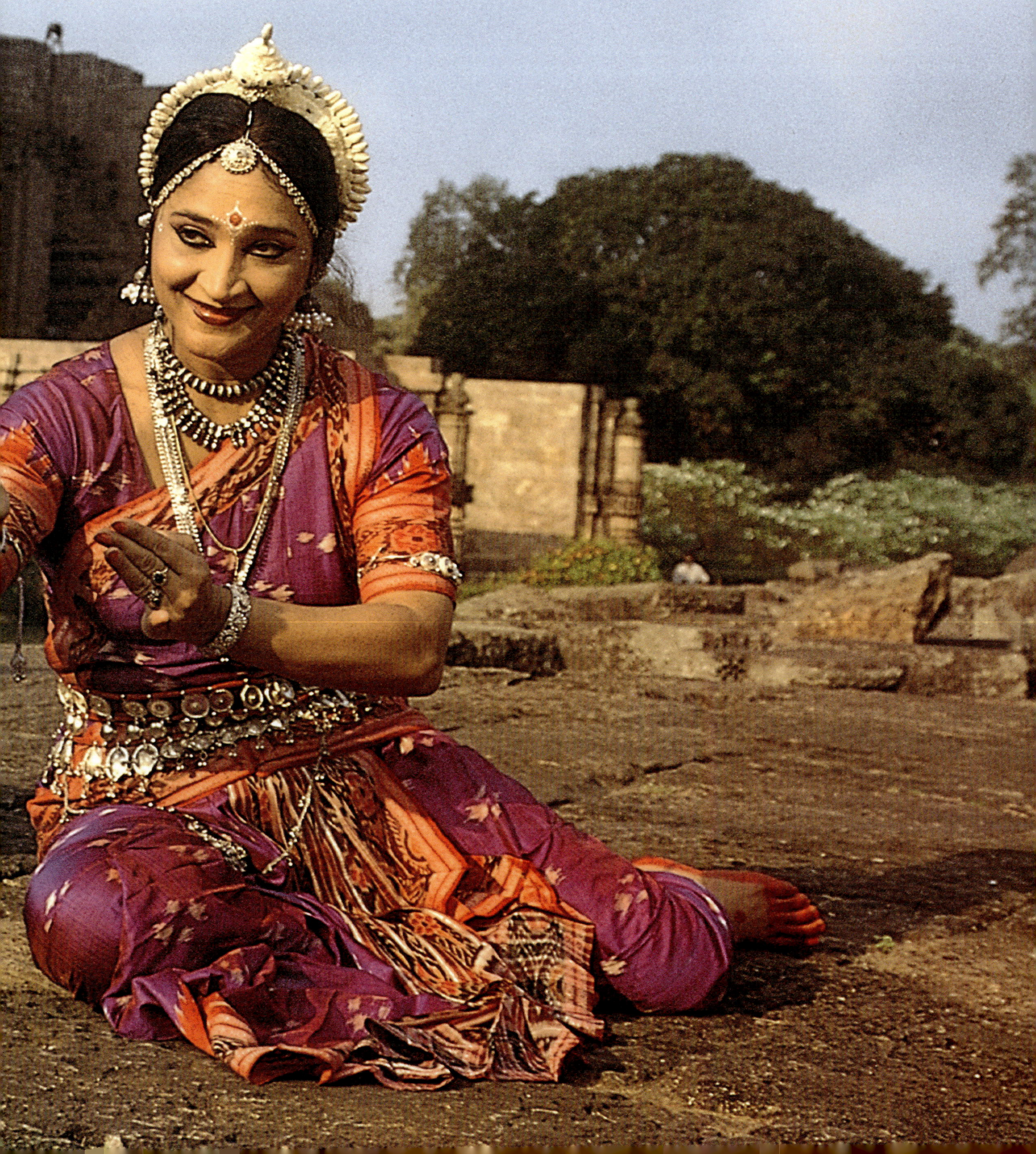

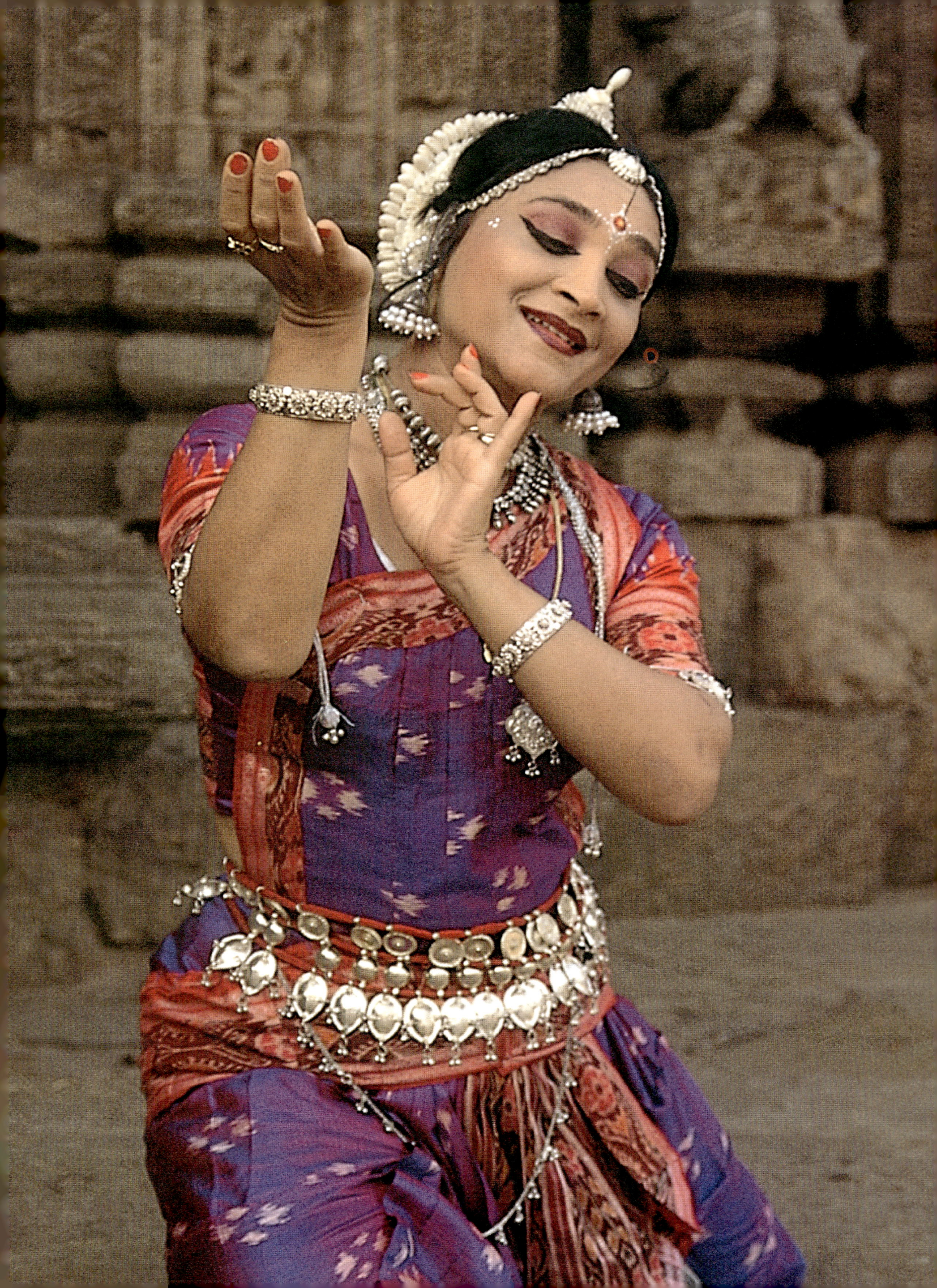

The vast treasure of the literature of Orissa relating to Odissi refers to the strength and purity, richness in tradition and authenticity of the art form. The ancient *Natya Shastra*, *Abhinaya Darpan* and Sharang Deva's *Sangeeta Ratnakar* have been the resources for various treatises related to the dance tradition of Orissa written at different periods. The unique features and techniques of Odissi are preserved and recorded in several manuscripts. They mention the style and the movement in dance, describe its *ragas*, *talas*, its instruments, and give detailed descriptions of the costume, ornaments and make-up which are still in practice. Most of the literature is in Sanskrit, written in Oriya script and is at least 300 years old. It was written on palm leaves and paper, and most of them were illustrated.

Of particular importance are the *Abhinaya Darpana Prakasha* by Jadunath Singha and the *Abhinaya Chandrika* by Maheswara Mahapatra. Apart from these, there are innumerable palm-leaf manuscripts pertaining to dance and music as practised in different periods in Orissa. Some of them have already been printed. These manuscripts are: *Natya Manorama, Sangeeta Narayana, Sangeeta Kalpalata, Sangeeta Sarani, Sangeeta Parijata and Geeta Parkash.* These texts are all based on the writings of sages like Bharata, Nandikeswara, Sarandeva, Kohala, Matanga and Narada. While quoting profusely the ancient masters, Oriya authors have also tried to incorporate the element of the regional technique.

The *Natya Shastra* of Bharata Muni, a 2000-year-old Sanskrit text, is the fundamental treatise on the performing arts in India. Theatre, music and Indian classical dance have their roots in the *Natya Shastra*, which provides a blueprint for India's performing arts prevalent today. Bharata Muni contends how the art of dance has two aspects—*tandava* and *lasya*. *Tandava* is the masculine or vigorous dance, whereas *lasya* is the feminine or soft form of the dance.

The Indian dance forms are often categorised as either *lokadharmi* or *natyadharmi*. The simple and down-to-earth dance forms, e.g., folk dances, come under *lokadharmi*, while those that are formal, contrived and defined by rules and principles belong to the *natyadharmi* tradition. Odissi is *natyadharmi* owing to its profoundity and the influence of the scriptures.

The *Natya Shastra* and later *Abhinaya Darpan* deal exhaustively with all aspects of the art of dance, particularly the technique. In contrast, classical dance is divided into *nritya* and *nritta*. *Nritta* is pure dance and the movements are performed for the sake of their own beauty and for the joy of dance. *Nritta* has two major constituents, *tala* or the time measure, and *laya* or the rhythm. *Nritya* is expressional or interpretative dance and its purpose is to convey a concept, theme or idea of *sahitya* (literature).

Left: A typical Odissi posture.

Following double spread: Depiction of abhinaya *in Odissi.*

Double spread pages 96-97: An Odissi dance posture depicting Krishna with his flute.

Page 98: Posture of playing the mardala.

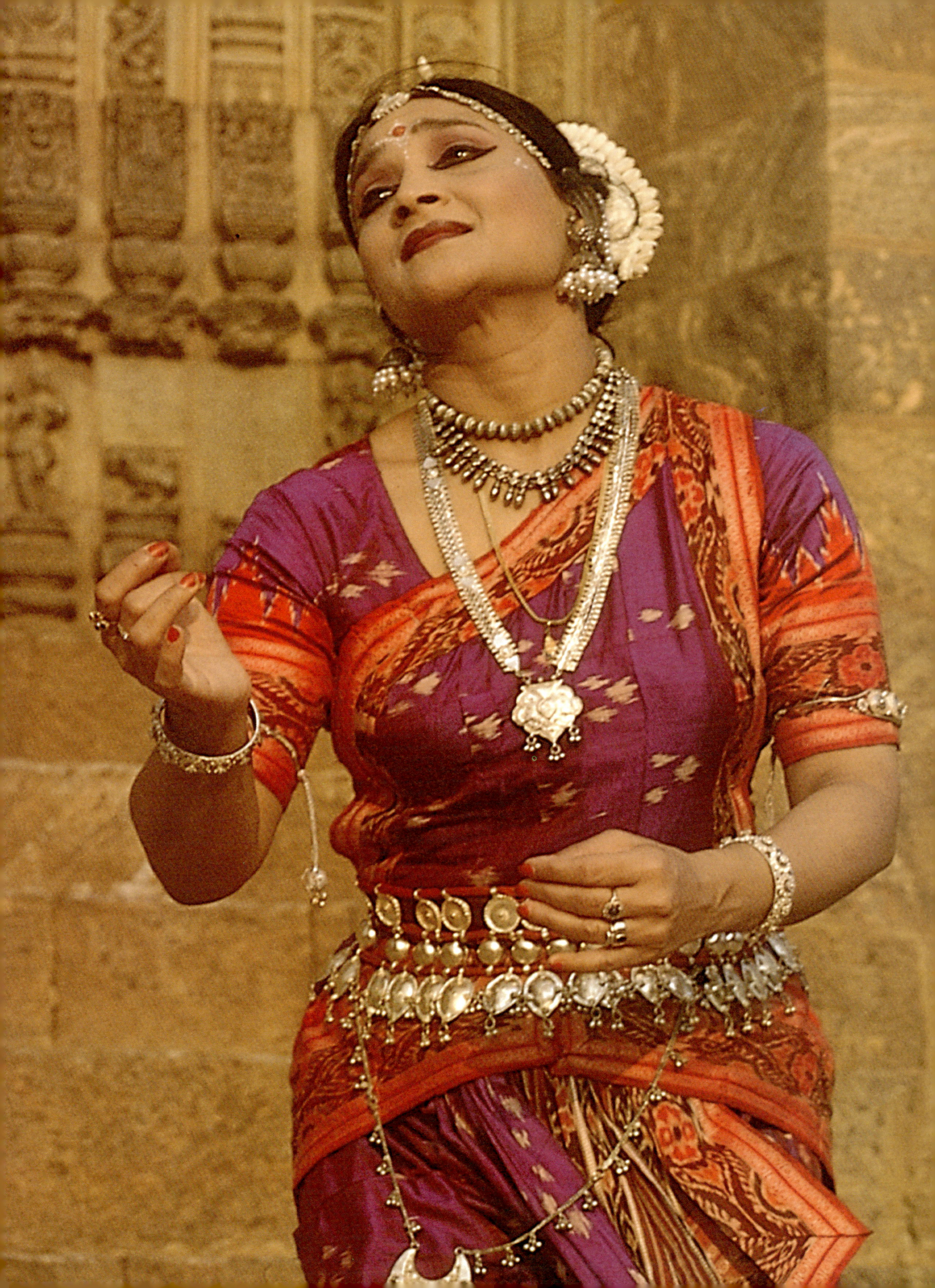

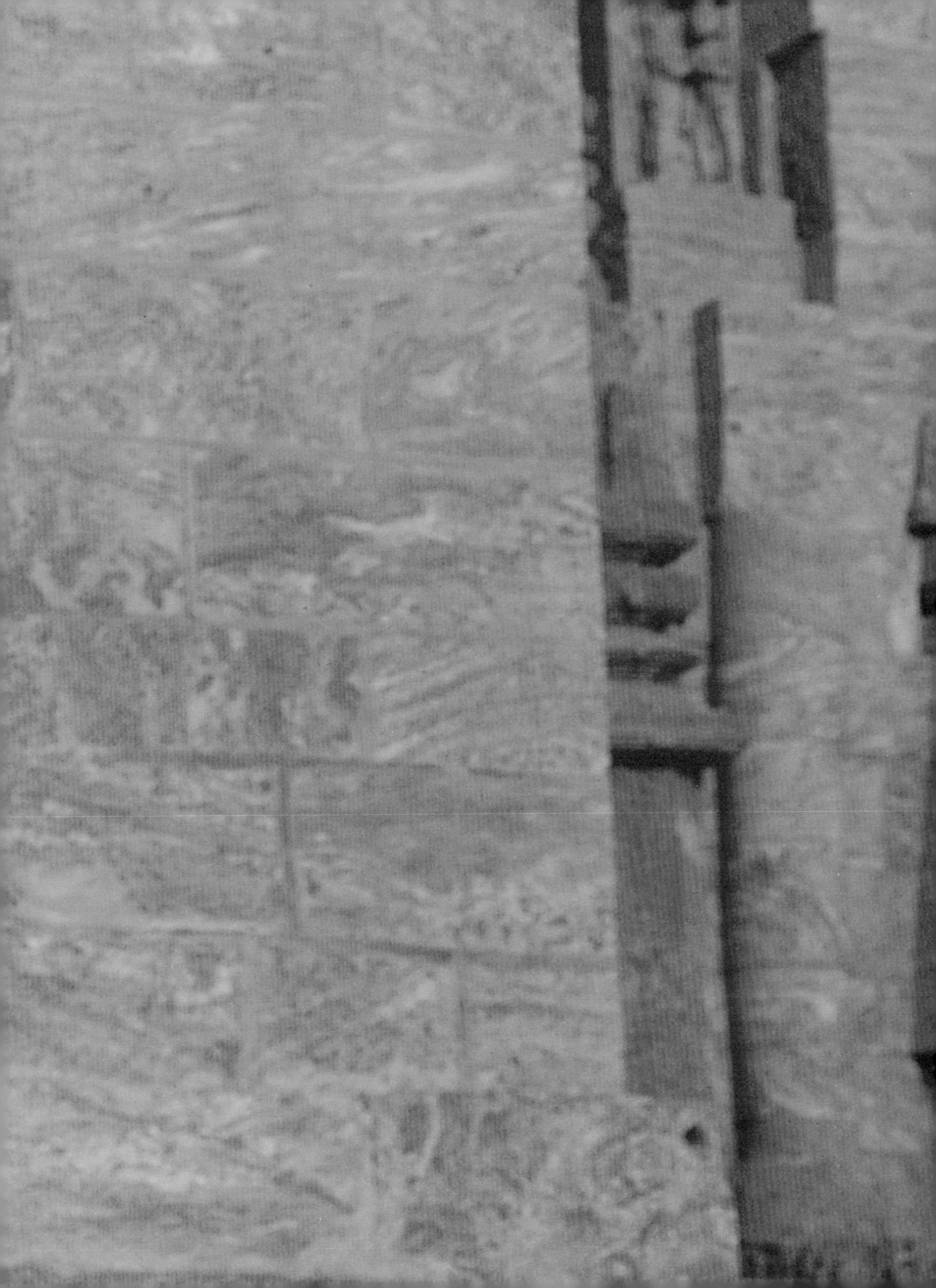

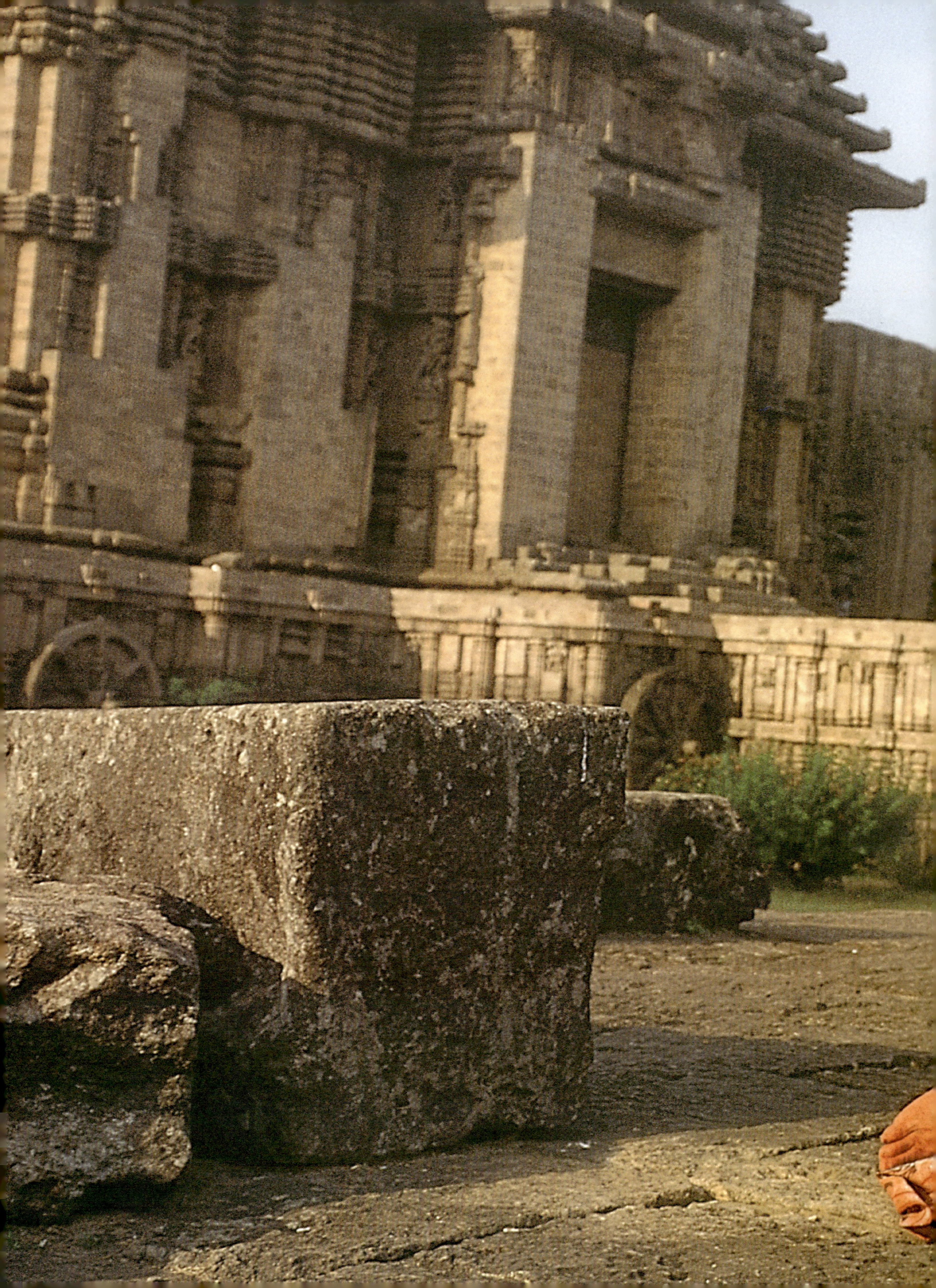

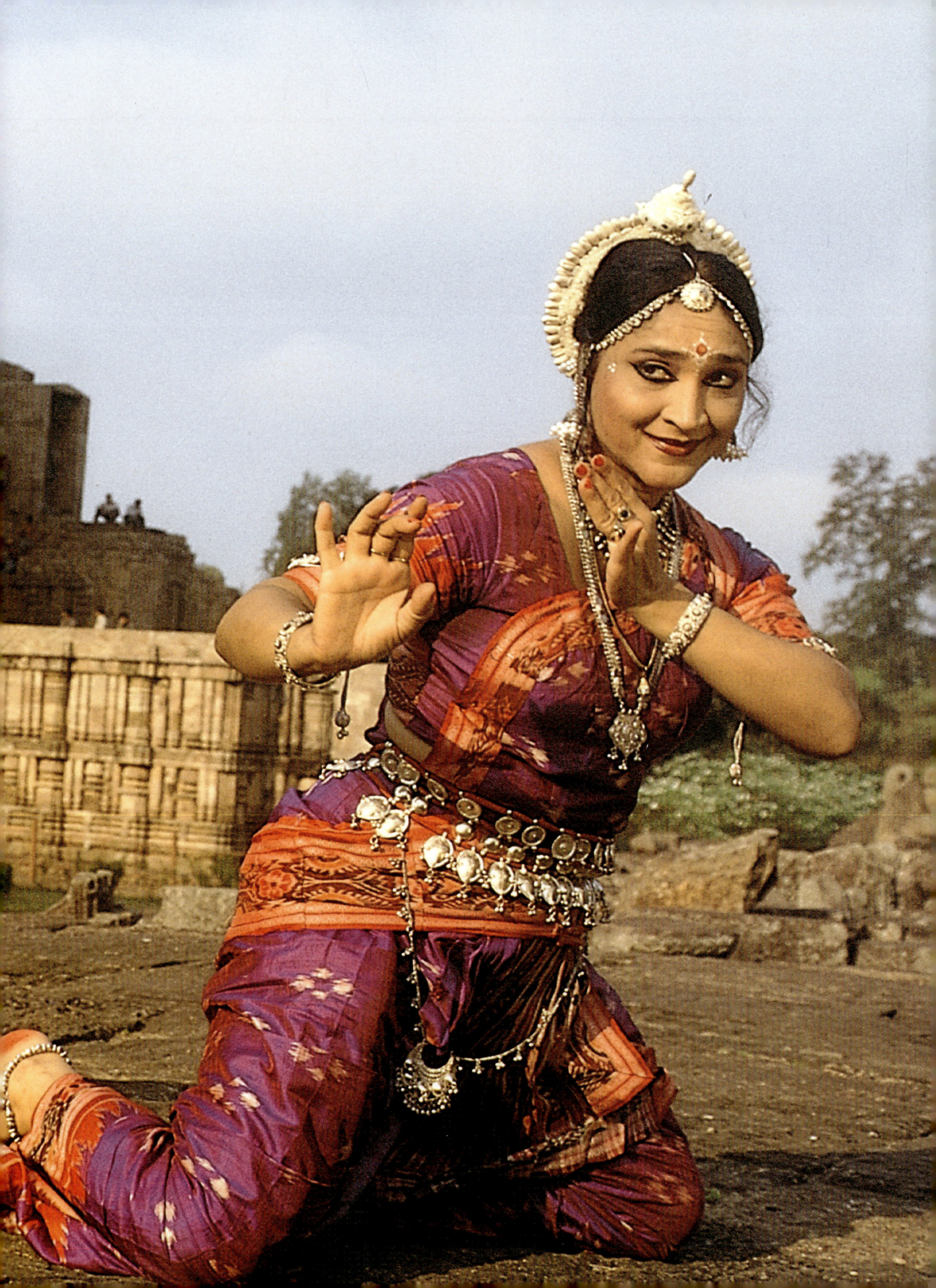

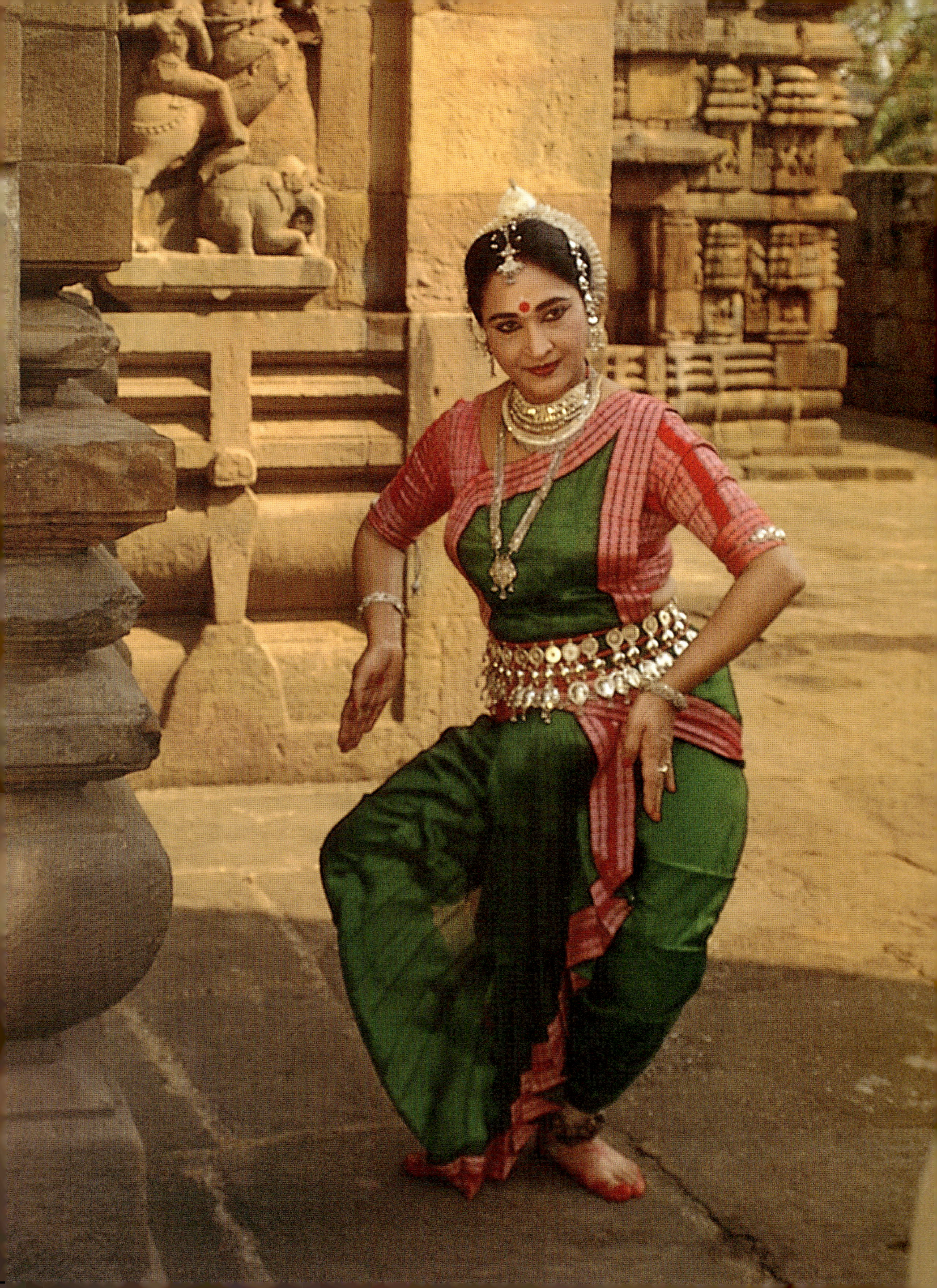

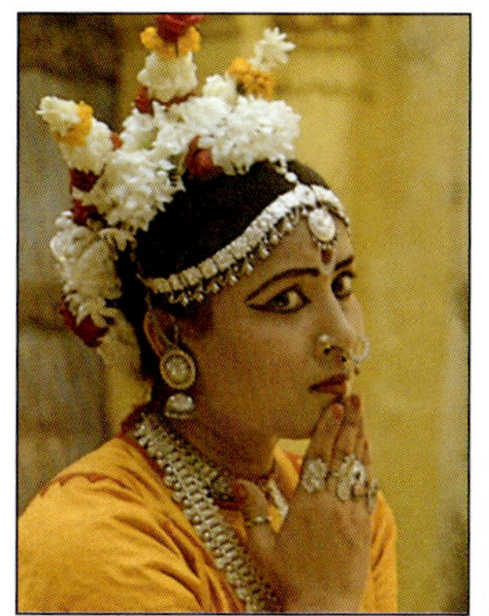

Abhinaya

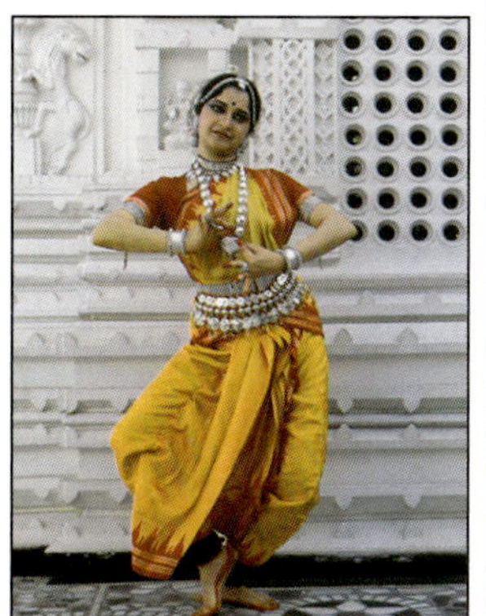

Bhangi

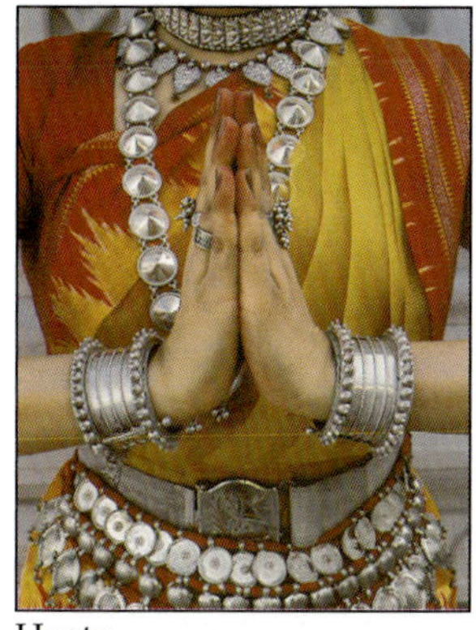

Hasta

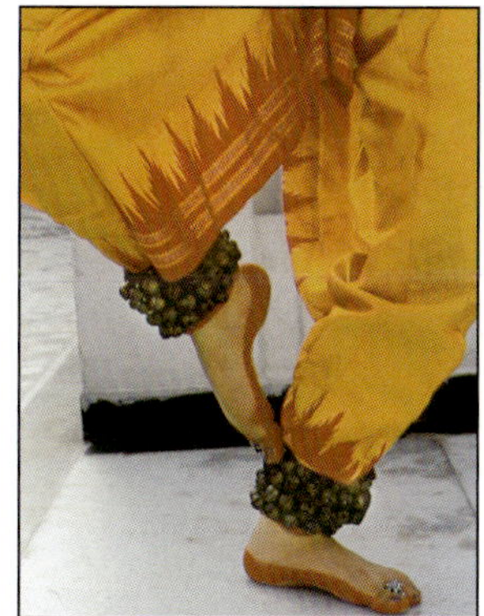

Pada bheda

Abhinaya can be translated as the transmission of expression, and it is also covered extensively in the *Natya Shastra*. In *nritya, abhinaya* is expressed through an elaborate system of facial expressions (*mukhabhinaya*), postures of the body (*bhangis*), hand gestures (*hastas*) and foot movement (*pada vinayas*) to convey the meaning of the story or the idea to the audience.

There are four forms of *abhinaya* which are blended in order to convey and project the expression to the audience, namely, *angika*, the movement and gestures of the body, which include facial expression, movements of each part of the body, particularly hand movements; *vachika*, voice and speech in the form of song or poetry; *sattwika*, play and interplay of moods, emotions and sentiments; and *aharya*, dress, adornment and make-up. All four types of *abhinaya* are represented in Odissi.

In Odissi, *abhinaya* is pure demonstration of an emotion contained in a song or lyric. Odissi stands out because of its distinctive and demure style of *abhinaya*. The *Geeta Govinda* forms the basis for one of the most important aspects of Odissi in which the song becomes a poem in action.

The tradition of songs, as we know it today in Orissa, perhaps began in the 12th century with the well-known *ashtapadis* of Jayadeva. The Sanskrit songs of the *Geeta Govinda* are in direct ancestral line of songs and musical poetry in Orissa. The *talas* and *ragas* are the same, so is the theme, and so the tendency to ornateness through assonances and alliterations. In medieval Oriya literature, the composers fixed the *tala* and *raga* of each song as in those of the *Geeta Govinda*. This has greatly helped maintain the purity of the style and continuance of the tradition.

The *Geeta Govinda* compositions are set in a slow tempo and the dancer gets complete scope to depict the emotion by gestures, glances and softer movements to reveal the entire meaning of the composition. The dancer, while portraying the *bhava*, brings out the myriad nuances of the *nayaka-nayika* concept of Hindu erotic psychology. Next to the *sringara rasa*, the songs used in this item deal with devotion or *bhakti rasa*. The *Dasavatara* composition of the *Geeta Govinda* is also one of the more popular pieces.

The Oriya songs are mostly medieval compositions of a large number of Vaishnavite poets and the theme obviously pertains to the relationship of Radha and Krishna. Among the composers, three dominate the field, Kavisurya Baladeva Ratha, Gopal Krishna Patnaik and Banamali Das. While Kavisurya is considered the most musical, Gopal Krishna the most poetic and Banamali the most devotional.

Dasavatara—*the ten incarnations of Lord Vishnu*

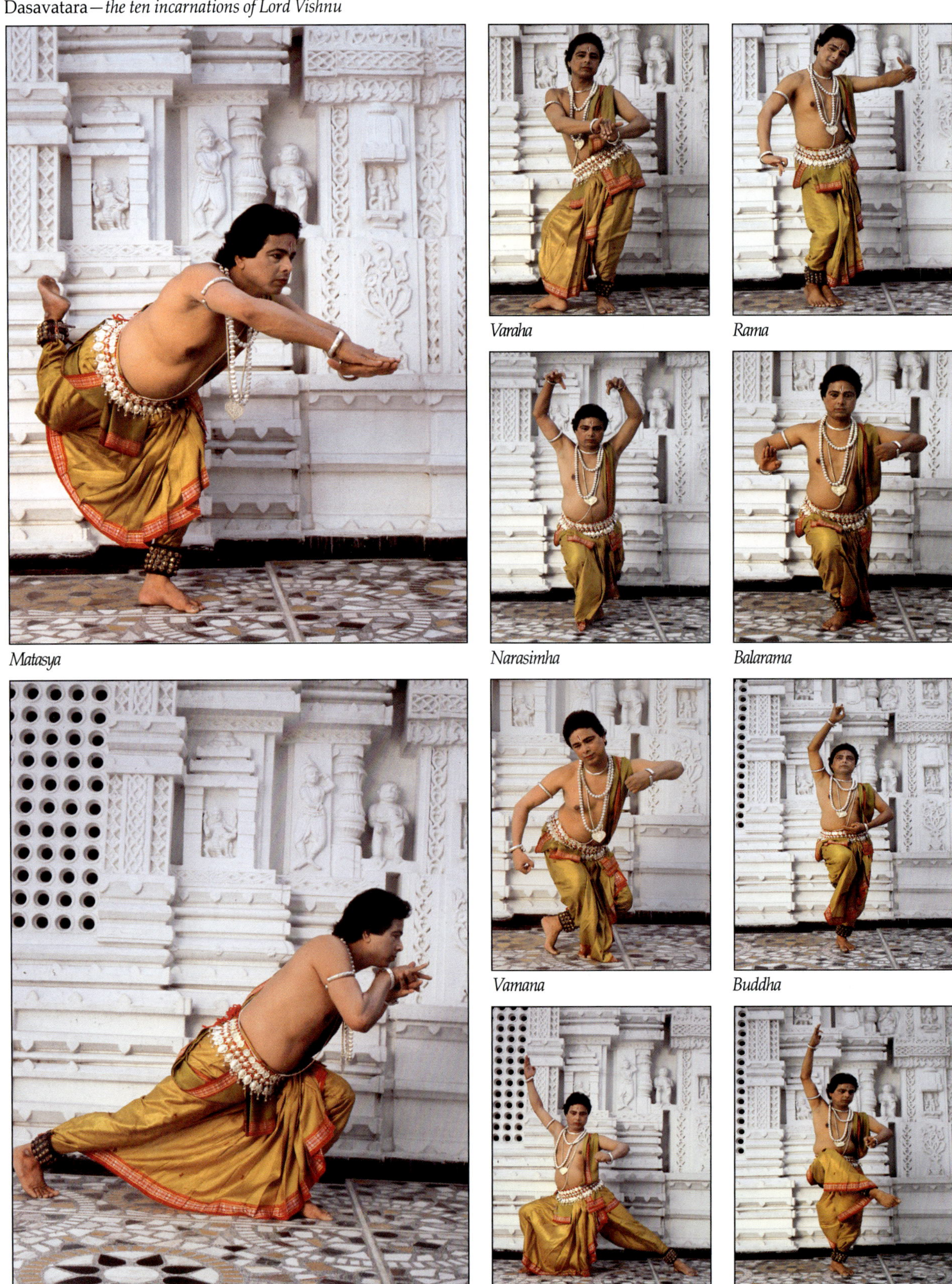

Matasya *Varaha* *Rama* *Narasimha* *Balarama* *Kurma* *Vamana* *Buddha* *Parashurama* *Kalki*

The *bhava-rasa* theory, given great importance in the *Natya Shastra*, is the heart of Indian classical dance, specially in the context of Odissi. *Bhava* can be explained as emotion. The literal meaning of *rasa* is juice, taste, flavour, and sweetness. *Rasa* creates the mood of a performance. The *bhava* and *rasa* of a skilled and talented dancer set the ambience of the performance and lead the audience to the idea or theme being conveyed by the dancer. *Bhava* and *rasa* together move and stir the audience and impart aesthetic enjoyment.

The nine *rasas* identified in the *Natya Shastra* are *sringara* (love), *veera* (valour), *karuna* (compassion), *adbhutam* (wonder), *bibhatsa* (repulsion), *hasya* (laughter), *bhaya* (fear), *raudra* (anger) and *shanta* (tranquillity). These *rasas* are not ordinary or transitory emotions but are 'universalised to reveal what is common in everyone's experience'.

A *shloka* of the *Natya Shastra* states:

यतो हस्तस्ततो दृष्टिर्यतो दृष्टिस्ततो मनः ।
यतो मनस्ततो भावो यतो भावस्ततो रसः ।।

Yato hastastato drishtiryato drishtirstato manaha I
Yato manstato bhavo yato bhavastato rasha II

— 37, *Abhinaya Darpana*

Where the hand goes, the eyes follow, where the eyes go, the mind follows,
And thus *bhava* is created and *rasa* will be born.

And creating and transmitting the *rasa* to the audience is the ultimate aim of any dancer.

Odissi reflects the iconography of Orissa as in the sculpturesque *tribanghi*, a three-bend posture, one of the most common in Odissi. There are numerous sculptures in the temples of Orissa in the *tribhangi* position. *Tribhangi* is a feminine posture and, as the name suggests, depicts three bends in the body. The other most commonly executed posture of Odissi is the *chauk*, considered to be the position of Lord Jagannath who is the all-pervading inspiration of the dance and of Orissa.

Subtle deflection of the hip is characteristic of Odissi. Movements are sometimes sharp, but mostly soft and lyrical. Many of the movements are in a half-sitting position, giving a sensuous touch. The numerous postures and styles portray specific moods.

It is primarily a *lasya* (feminine) dance although some elements of *tandava* (masculine) form part of its technique. This vigorous *tandava* element is probably due to the influence of the Shaivite school of dancing. Female figures in *tandava* attitude can be seen in the temples of Mukteshwar and Jagannath.

Nritta and *nritya* are given equal representation in the Odissi repertoire. In *nritta*, or pure dance, great importance is given to balance and harmony and the stylised movements which convey the pure techniques of the dance form. In *nritya*, emotions and sentiments are expressed through the eyes, facial expressions and *hasta mudra* to convey and portray various moods or *bhava* and, more importantly, to elicit an emotional response in the audience, that is, to evoke *rasa*.

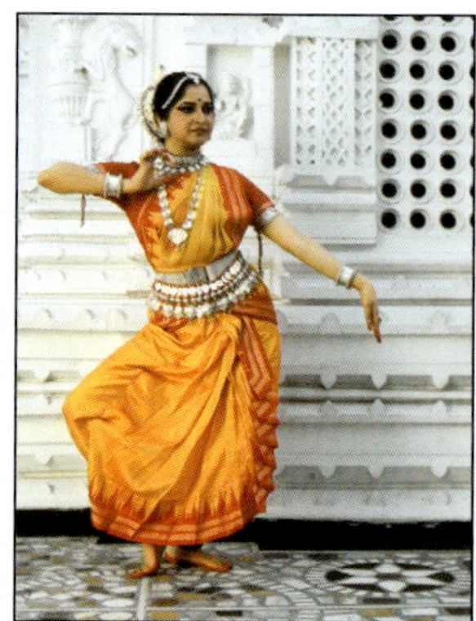

Lasya

Technique

Odissi is full of sculpturesque poses known as *bhangis*. In all its movements, an attempt is always made to elicit grace and charm. The technique of Odissi dance consists of: *pada bheda*, or positions of the feet; *bhumi*, or lines in which a dancer moves on the stage; *chari*, or the different kinds of steps; *bhramari*, the whirling movements in dance; *bhangi*, the basic poses and movements of *nritta; hasta mudras* or gesture language which endeavours to convey the meaning of the idea to be portrayed.

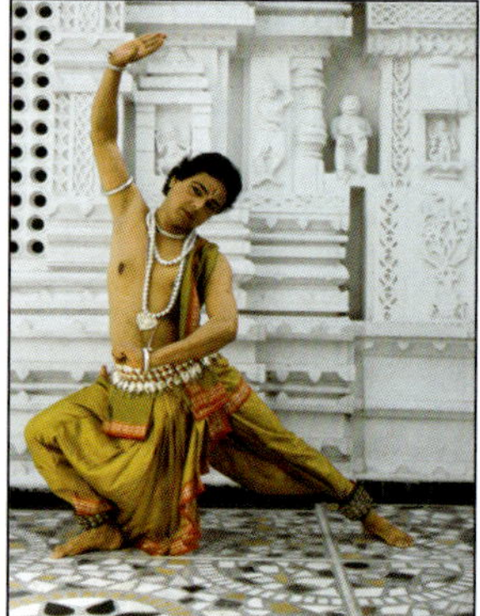

Tandava

One of the most common and fundamental positions of Odissi is the *chauk*. In this squatting position, the dancer's weight is evenly distributed, making the thighs almost horizontal, while the arms are kept to the sides and the front. The other is the *tribhangi,* which is created by three *bhanga* (body bends), in which the head, torso and hips are deflected and which is commonly used in Odissi dance in a variety of permutations and combinations. It is not only difficult to execute but also calls for immense restraint and finesse.

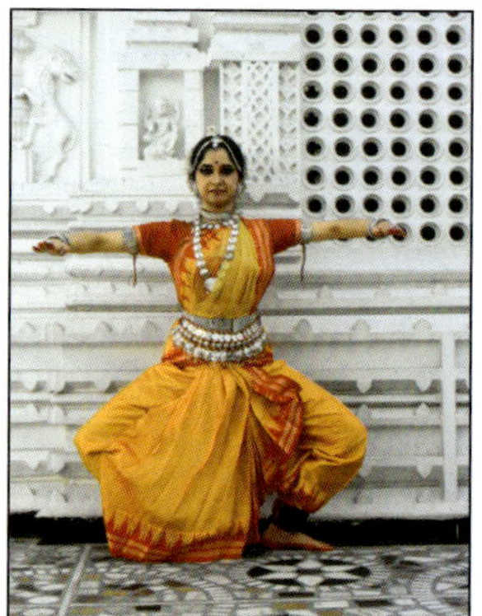

Chauk

According to the *Abhinaya Chandrika*, the treatise on Odissi dance written in the 15th century, there are four basic *pada bhedas* or positions of the feet, that are fundamental to Odissi: *stambhapada, kumbhapada, dhanupada* and *mahapada*. *Stambhapada* and *kumbhapada* are the same as *samapada* and *ayata mandalapada*, described in the *Abhinaya Darpana*. The author also refers to *padas* mentioned in the *Sangeeta Ratnakar* of Sharang Deva. They are *sama, suchi, ghatita, agratala sanchara, mardita, agraga, parsvaga* and *samakunchana* (*kunchita*). The *vismapada* he mentions is the same as *traisrpada* of the *Natya Shastra*.

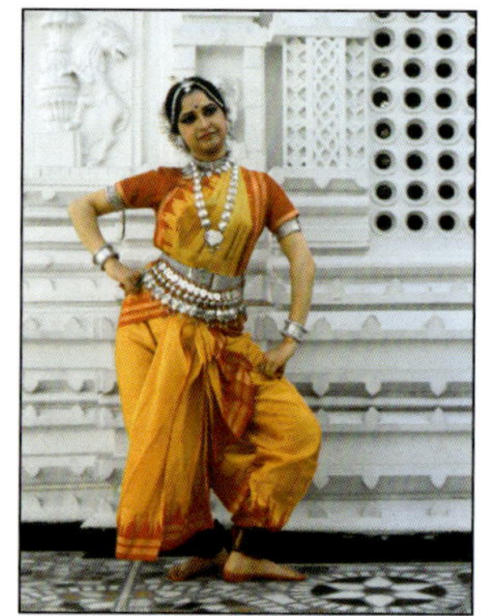

Tribhangi

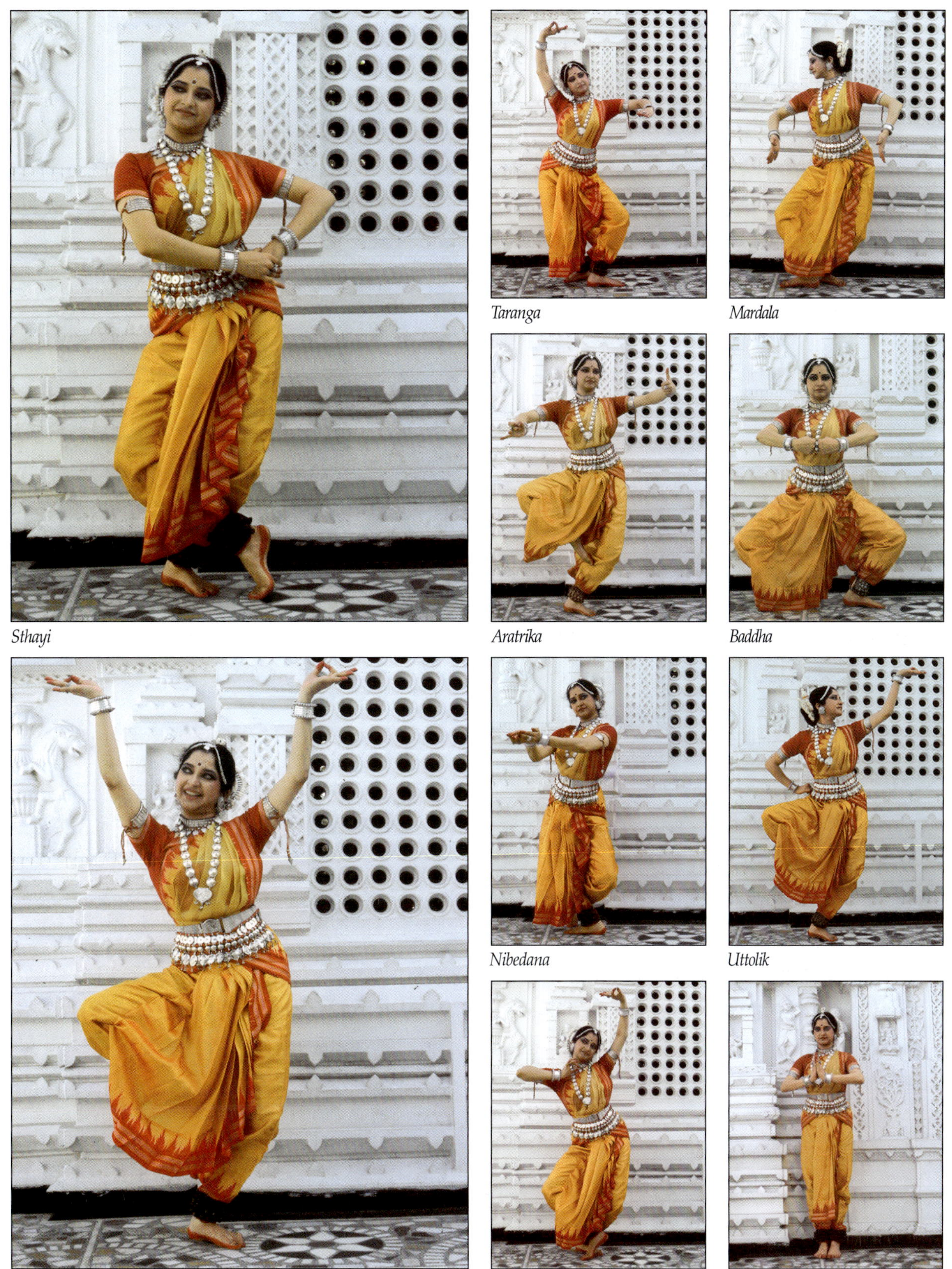
Sthayi

Taranga

Mardala

Aratrika

Baddha

Kshipta

Nibedana

Uttolik

Abhimana

Pranata

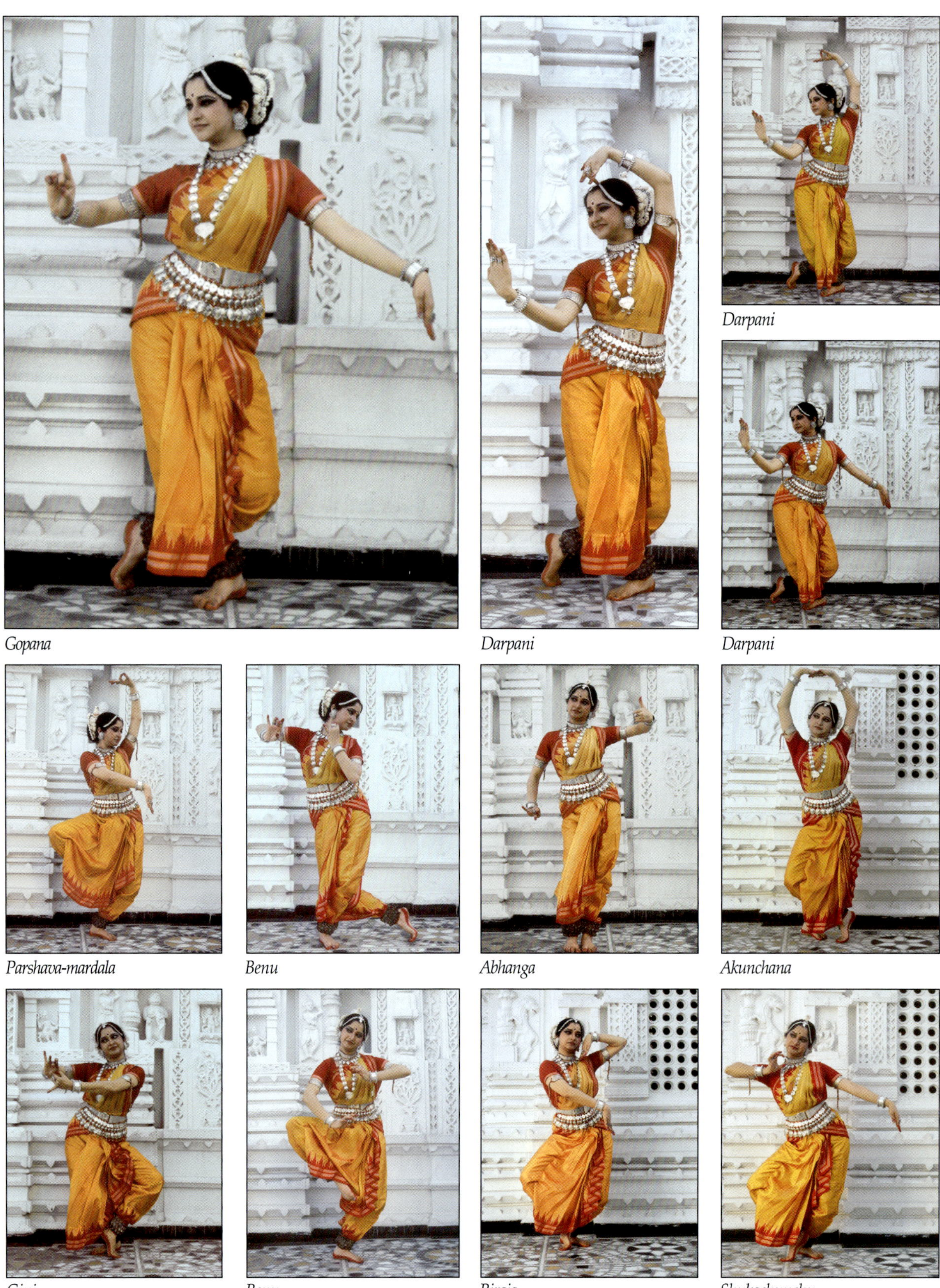

Gopana

Darpani

Darpani

Darpani

Parshava-mardala

Benu

Abhanga

Akunchana

Gini

Benu

Biraja

Shukachunchu

The traditional positions of the feet are known as *rekhapada, ashrtapada, nupurapada,* to name a few.

The heels play an important part and there is one movement in which the dancer moves on the heels alone. This is done during the ending of a dance piece and always precedes *tihai*, i.e., the time cycle repeated three times or final beat. In this movement, the dancer jumps forward and moves on the heels round his person or recedes to take a final position. Related to *pada bhedas* are the *bhumis,* which are the lines of movement of a dancer when performing. There are eight *bhumis* mentioned in the *Abhinaya Chandrika*—*sama, visama, padma, trikonaka, svastika, chakra, vatula* and *chaturasra* or *chauka*. The most famous of these is the *chauka* in which the dancer moves in an imaginary square.

The actual steps taken by the dancer are known as *charis.* In Odissi, the *charis* listed in the *Abhinaya Darpana* of Nandikeswara are strictly followed and they are: *chalana, chankramana, sarana, begini, kuttana, luthita* and *visama.*

When the basic movements of the dance are combined with the principal body positions, these are known as *belis,* of which there are eight—*utha, baitha, thia, chali, burha, bhasa, bhaunri* and *pali*. For instance:

Utha is rising with a jump from a sitting position.

Baitha or *utaplavana* is a semi-seated pose with one knee resting on the ground position.

Thia is a standing position.

Chali is rhythmic gait and gyrating movement.

Burha is a pose depicting bliss. It is a beautiful *tribhangi* pose with arms arched above the head and fingertips touching.

Bhasa is the diagonal swing of the torso (*antibhanga*) from side to side, knees bent, and arms moving rhythmically to each side.

Bhaunri or *bhramari* is a whirling movement or a spin. There are many kinds of *bhaunri* in Odissi. *Ekapada bhramari* is a pivot on one foot and *chakra bhramari* is a fast revolving movement with one foot hitting the ground.

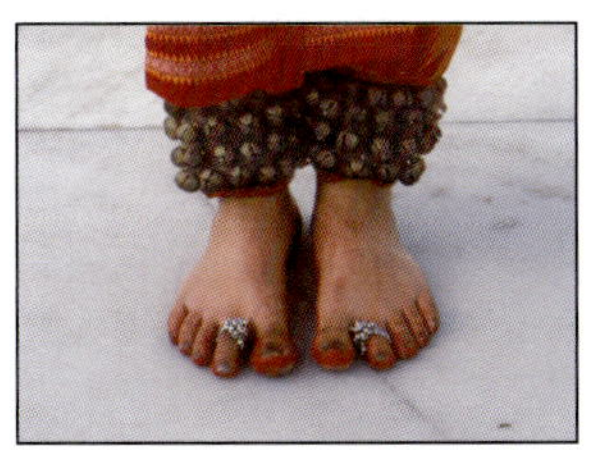

Stambhapada

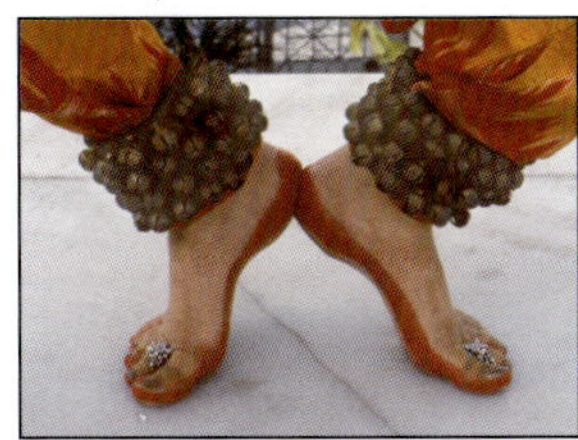

Kumbhapada

Then there are *kunchita* and *anga bhramaris*. All these adhere to the *Abhinaya Darpana*. Out of these, the most dominating in Odissi is *ekapada bhramari*. This is performed in the *chauka* position both in clockwise and anti-clockwise movements.

Hand gestures or *hasta mudras* used for interpreting are a unique feature of Indian classical dance. This hand gesture language has a rich vocabulary, which is able to interpret different ideas, characters and situations in dance. In *nritya* or interpretative dance, expression is achieved through what can be called the poetic language of the hands or *hasta mudras. Nritta hastas* are used for decorative effect whereas *nritya hastas* are used to convey meaning. Some of these are based on the *Natya Shastra* and *Abhinaya Darpana,* but the typical *hastas* mentioned in Oriya scriptures are peculiar to Odissi.

In *nritya* the *hastas* serve as a gesture language, which endeavours to convey the meaning of the idea to be portrayed. In this connection, the *Abhinaya Darpana* clearly states: '*Hastenartham Pradarshayet*' (the vocabulary of the *hastas*). Corresponding to the *hastas* involved, emotions and sentiments are also expressed through the eyes. In Bharata's *Natya Shastra*, Nandikeswara's *Abhinaya Darpana,* Sharang Deva's Sangeeta *Ratnakar*, Dhananjaya's *Dasarupaka* and in many other similar texts, *hastas* have been elaborately defined and their usage precisely indicated. In Odissi, the *hastas* constitute as essential a part of the technique as in the case of Bharatnatyam and Kathakali.

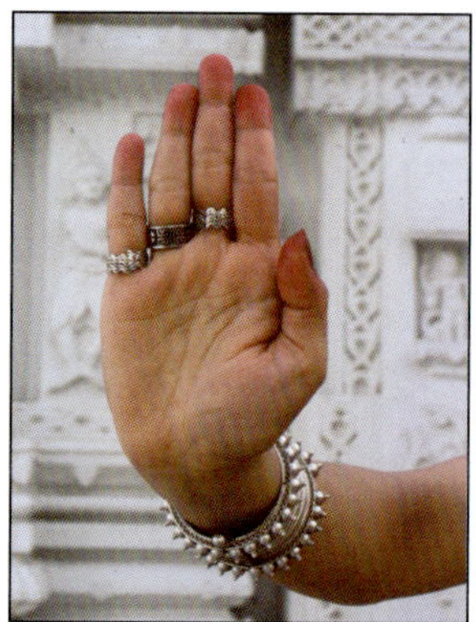
Pataka

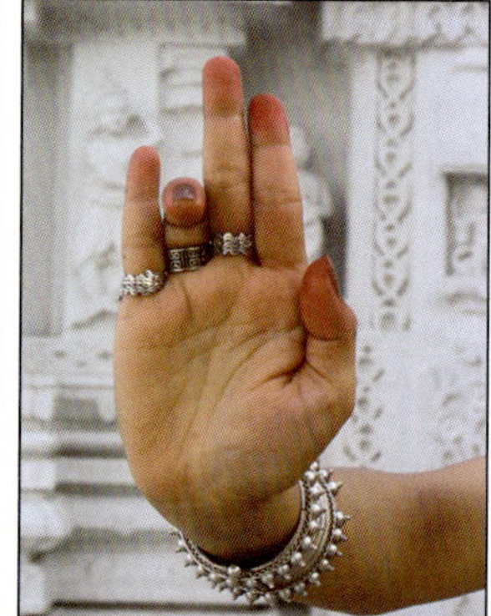
Tripataka

Hand Gestures

The hand gestures as described in Nandikeswara's *Abhinaya Darpana* are as follow:

Asamyuta Hasta—Single Hands

1. *Pataka* (flag): The palm is stretched, the thumb is bent close to the hand while all the fingers are opened out straight and close together.

Application: It is used in the beginning and end of *natya*. This hand represents Indra's flagstaff and is a sign of victory. It indicates divine assurance and grace. It is used for saying 'I am', 'me', 'here', waves, cloud, river, pool, night, wind, bosom, horse, lying down, moonlight, strong sunlight, forcing open doors, benediction, aversion, ideal king, addressing a person, going forward, holding a sword, month, year, rainy day and cleaning as with a broom.

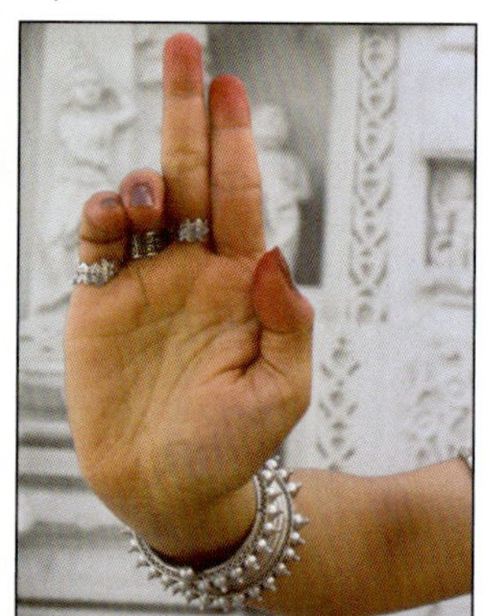
Ardha-pataka

2. *Tripataka*: It is a flag with three fingers pose. The third finger of the *pataka* hand is bent *down* at the middle joint.

Application: It is used to represent a crown, invocation, descent of the gods or *avatara*, a god, or the gods in heaven (held above the head, or crossed). It is used for holding weapons or symbols of the god, Indra, i.e., *vajra*, (thunderbolt); to apply sacred marks to the forehead and to wipe away tears (with the third finger), to indicate going, the feet (palm down), tree,

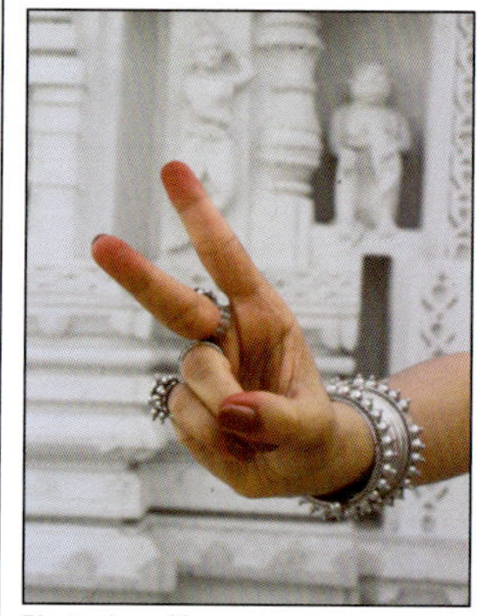
Kartari-mukha

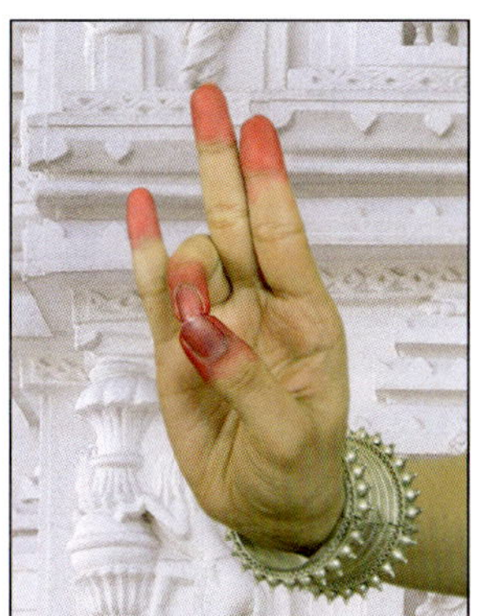
Mayura

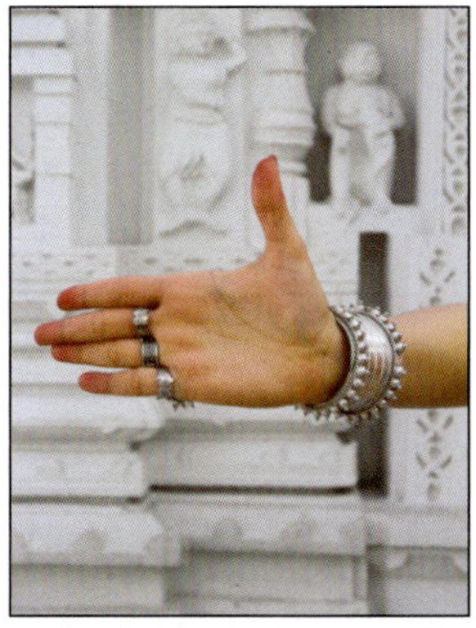
Ardha-chandra

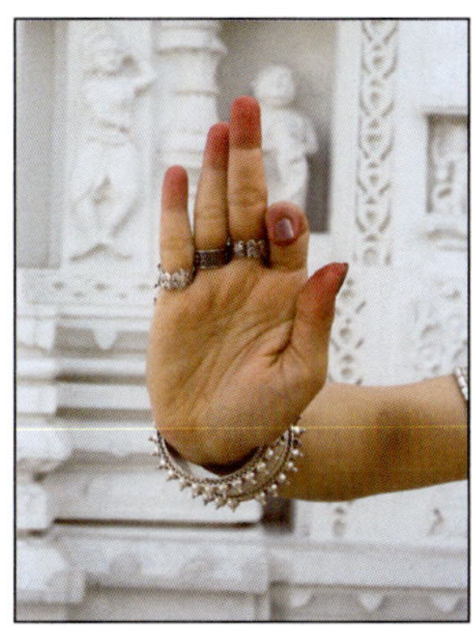
Arala

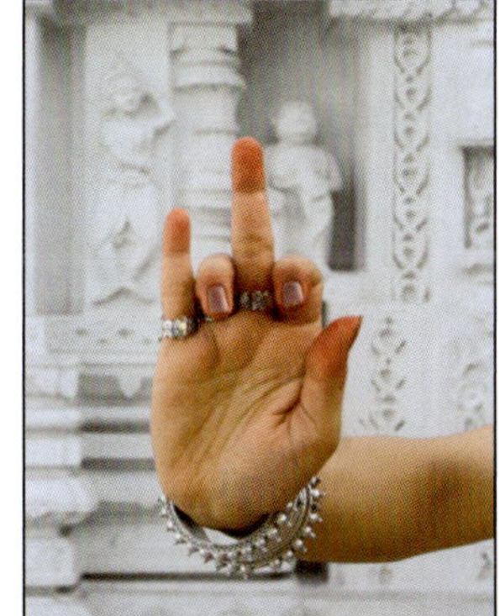
Sukatunda

arrow-shaft, lightning, fire, a lamp, *ketaki* flower, a pigeon, an arrow and turning around.

3. *Ardha-pataka* (half flag): If the little finger of the *tripataka* hand is bent, the *hasta* is called *ardha-pataka*.

Application: It is used to denote leaves, a board or a slab for writing or painting, river bank, saying 'two things', knife, banner, tower and horn.

4. *Kartari-mukha* (scissors' mouth): The first and second fingers of the *ardha-pataka* hand are separated, the first being extended backward.

Application: It is used to denote the separation of a man and a woman in love, overturning or opposition, plundering, corner of an eye, death, estrangement, lightening, sleeping alone, falling and weeping, going, showing the way, steps of walking, horns of an animal, hypocrisy, creeper.

5. *Mayura* (peacock): The third finger of the *tripataka* hand is joined to the thumb and the other fingers are stretched.

Application: It is used to represent the peacock and its neck, a creeper, a bird, vomiting, removing as well as plaiting the hair, ornamental mark on the forehead (*tilak*), scattering (agitating), river water, discussing scriptures, a famous thing.

6. *Ardha-chandra* (half moon): The thumb of the *pataka* hand is extended to form an angle with the hand.

Application: It is used to represent the moon on the eighth day of the dark fortnight, a hand seizing the throat, a spear, consecration of an image, a dining plate, origin, waist, musing, meditation, prayers, touching limbs, greeting by the common people, to slay (diagonal downward movement), battle axe, the body, hips, face, mirror, beating time, resting the cheek on the hand, ear of an elephant, mirror. Making *ardha-chandra* with both hands, the right upward and the left downward is called *abhaya mudra*, the gesture of Shiva, indicating fearlessness and hope.

7. *Arala* (bent): The first finger of the *pataka* hand is curved and the other fingers are stretched out.

Application: It represents drinking poison, nectar, violent winds, gathering the hair, calling anyone, sweet smell, arranging patterns or flowers on the ground.

8. *Sukatunda* (parrot's head): In the *arala hasta* when the third finger is bent at the middle joint, it is called *Sukatunda*.

Application: It represents shooting an arrow, throwing a spear, remembering one's abode, speaking of mystic things and violent mood.

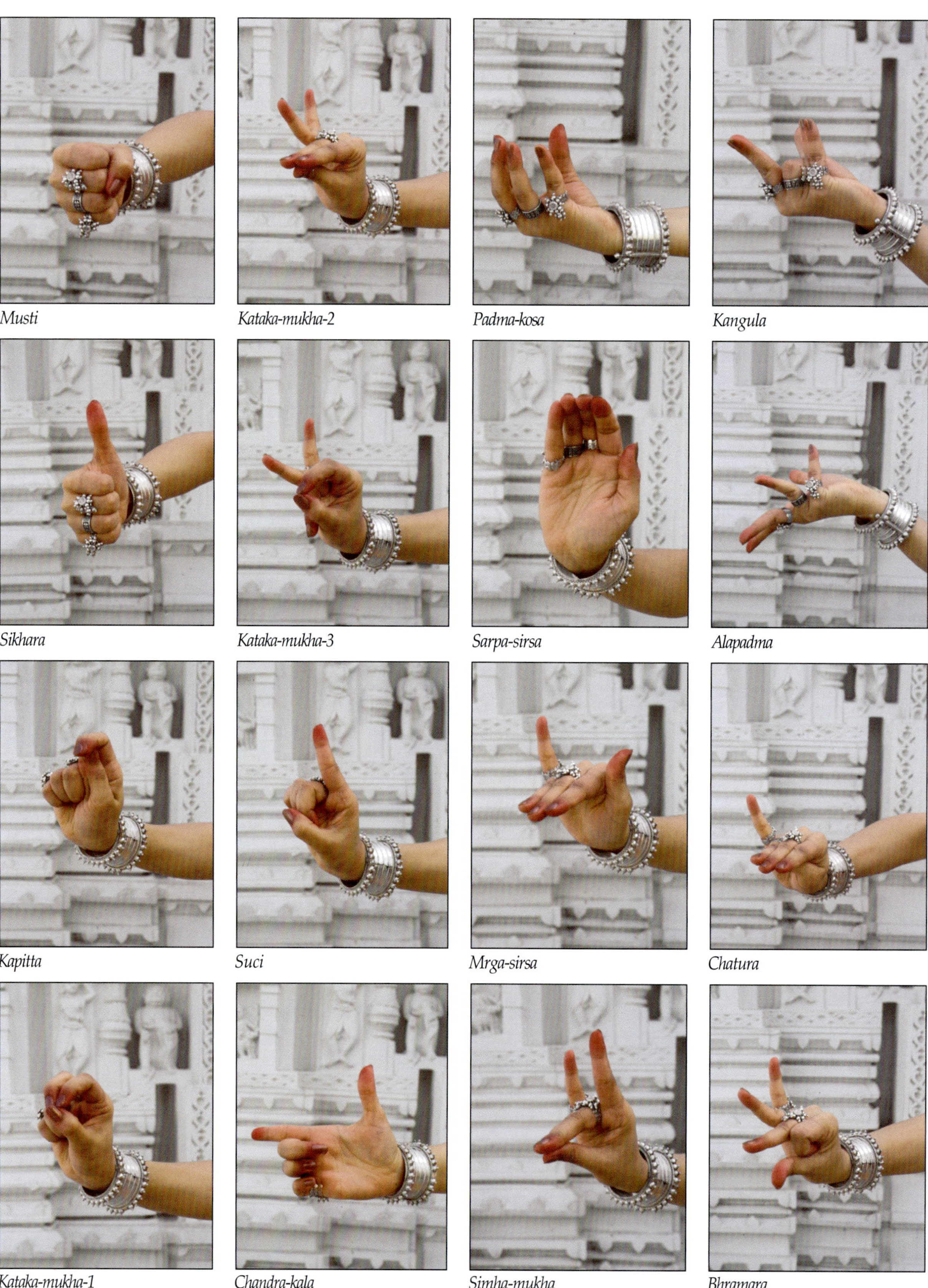

Musti | Kataka-mukha-2 | Padma-kosa | Kangula

Sikhara | Kataka-mukha-3 | Sarpa-sirsa | Alapadma

Kapitta | Suci | Mrga-sirsa | Chatura

Kataka-mukha-1 | Chandra-kala | Simha-mukha | Bhramara

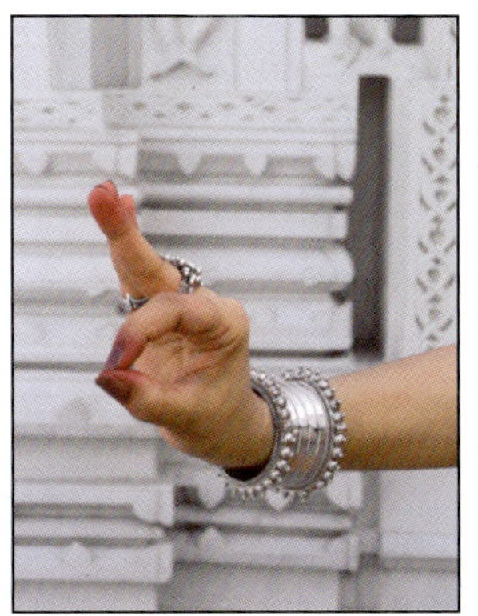
Hamsasya

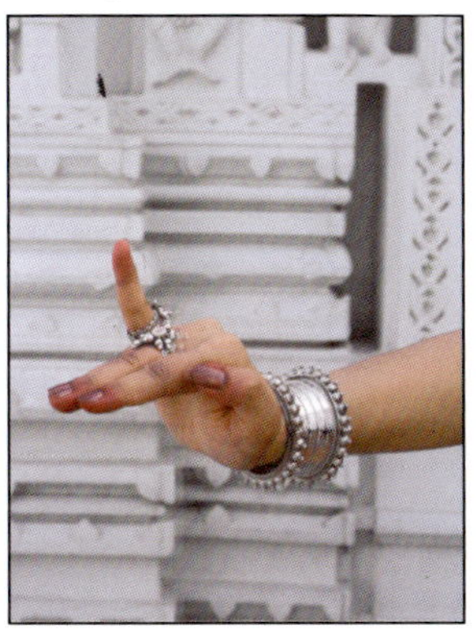
Hamsa-paksa

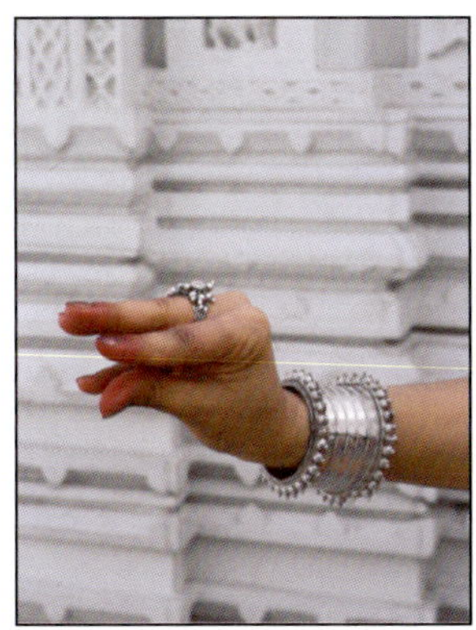
Samdamsa-1

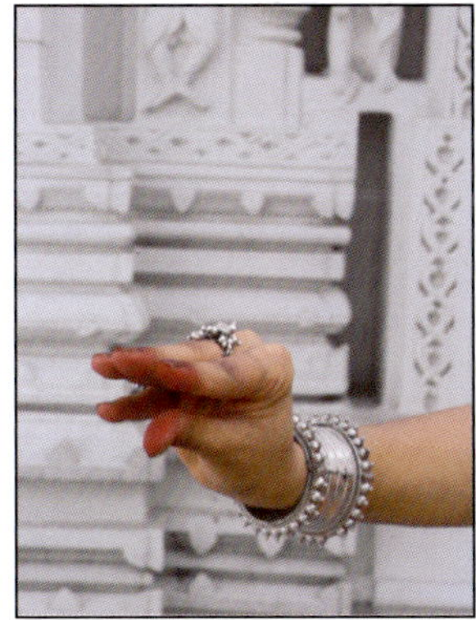
Samdamsa-2

9. *Musti* (fist): All the four fingers are closed into the palm, and the thumb is bent over them.

Application: It represents strength and steadiness, grasping one's hair, holding things, fighting mood or threatening like a wrestler.

10. *Sikhara* (peak or summit): The thumb of the *musti* hand is extended or raised.

Application: It denotes armour or Kamadeva—God of Love, to hold the bow, pillar, certainty, showing the lips, something entering, tooth, questioning, *shivalinga*, saying 'no', recollection, untying the girdle, embrace, sounding a bell.

11. *Kapitta* (bird): In this hand gesture, the forefinger of the *sikhara* hand is bent over the thumb and the other fingers closed in the palm.

Application: It represents Lakshmi—Goddess of Wealth, Saraswati—Goddess of Knowledge, holding symbols, milking cows, applying collyrium, holding flowers in a mood of romance, holding a veil or the end of a robe, offering incense or light, churning, holding flower garlands.

12. *Kataka-mukha* (opening a link): The third and fourth fingers of the *kapitta* hand are raised and the middle finger remains bent.

Application: It represents picking and collecting flowers, holding a necklace or a flower garland, drawing the middle of the bow, offering betel leaves, preparing the paste of *sandal* or musk, applying perfume, speaking and glancing, a woman, flower-tipped arrows of Kamadeva—God of Love, arranging ornaments, holding a *veena* (lute), a flute, conversation, addressing the beloved.

13. *Suci* : The first finger of the *kataka-mukha* hand is raised, and the thumb joined to the tip of the middle finger.

Application: It represents number 'one', the Supreme Soul, one hundred, the sun, a city, the world, saying 'like that', in the sense of solitude, threatening, becoming thin, a rod, body, astonishment, a braid of hair, an umbrella, capability, hairs, beating the drum, the potter's wheel, consideration and the decline of the day.

14. *Chandra-kala* (crescent moon): The thumb of the *suci* hand is stretched so that the first finger and thumb form the crescent moon.

Application: It represents the moon, the face, crown of Shiva, Ganga, a cudgel, tusks of an elephant or a boar.

15. *Padma-kosa* (lotus bud): The fingertips are brought close together without touching while the palm is hollowed to form the lotus bud.

Application: It represents fruits, breasts of a woman, a circular movement, ball, cooking pot, taking meals, flower bud, scattering flowers, cluster of flowers, to worship Shiva with lotus flowers, bell, an anthill and an egg.

16. *Sarpa-sirsa* (snake's head): The *pataka* hand is curved and the palm is hollowed to form a snake's head.

Application: It represents sandal-paste, a serpent, sprinkling water, water offering to gods, arms of a wrestler.

17. *Mrga-sirsa* (dear head): The little finger and thumb of the *sarpa-sirsa* hand are raised and separated from the other fingers.

Application: It denotes a woman, cheek, wheel, fear, quarrel, costume, *tilak* on the forehead, deer, flute of Krishna, stepping and calling the beloved.

18. *Simha-mukha* (lion-face): The tips of the middle and third fingers are joined to the thumb, and the other fingers are raised.

Application: It represents offering to the sacred fire, a hare, an elephant, lotus garland, face of a lion, salvation (*moksha*), drawing bow of Kamadeva.

19. *Kangula* (a tail): The third finger of the *padma-kosa* hand is bent toward the palm and the other fingers are raised.

Application: It is used to represent a small fruit and small things, jewels and bells, a partridge, a betel nut tree, a water lily, a *cataka* bird, a coconut, bee in lotus.

20. *Alapadma* (full-blown lotus): All the fingers are separated with a slight twisting movement beginning with the little finger.

Application: It represents a lotus in full bloom, circular movement, breasts, full moon, beauty, hair knot, a tower, a village, height, anger, a lake, praise.

21. *Chatura* (clever): The thumb of the *mrga-sirsa* hand is placed at the base of the third finger.

Application: It denotes musk, a little, metals like gold, wet, sorrow, aesthetics, pleasure, stepping slowly, to show cleverness of eye, shame, lotus petal, sidelong glance, sufficiency, seat, the number 'four', the four *Vedas*, Brahma—the four-faced god, oil and ghee.

22. *Bhramara* (bee): When the thumb and middle finger touch, the first finger is bent and the other fingers are raised and separated.

Application: It stands for a bee (with shaking movement), crane, flying creatures, vow of silence, holy bath (the tip of the nose held between the thumb and the middle finger), earring.

23. *Hamsasya* (swan-face): The forefinger touches the thumb and the other fingers are separated and raised.

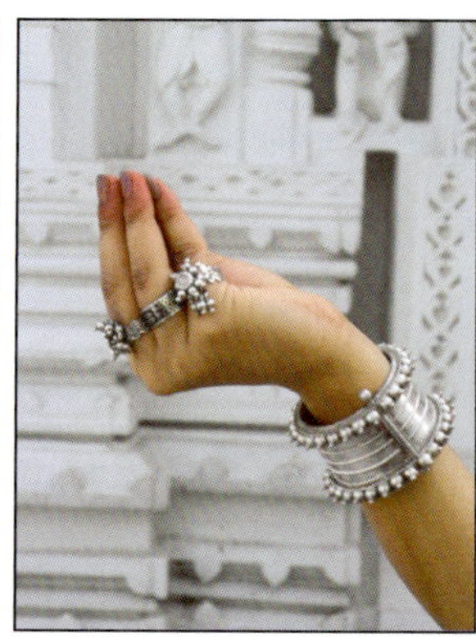

Mukula

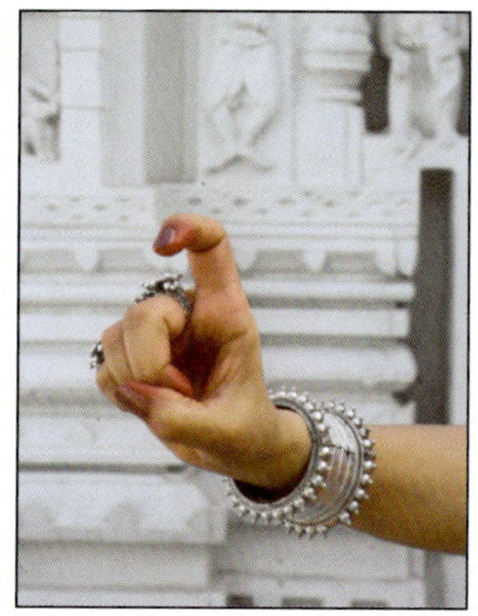

Tamra-cuda

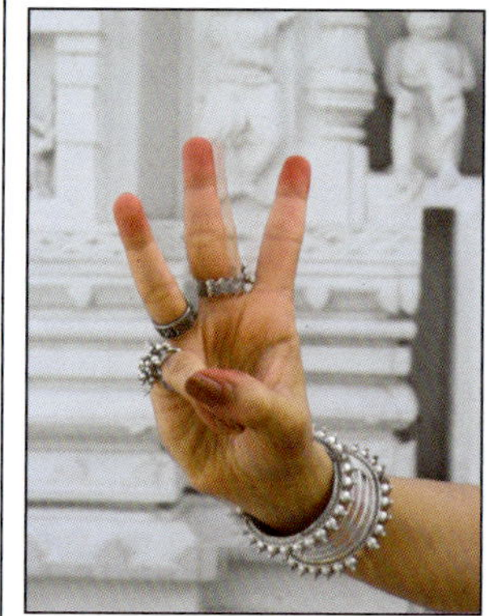

Trishula

Application: It represents blessings, instruction in ritual, tying with thread, pearls, pushing forward the wick of a lamp, a jasmine, the act of painting, swan, purity, meditation, speaking, offering things, a gem, a drop of water, affection, compassion, lightness, softness, insect (with tips of fingers throbbing).

24. *Hamsa-paksa* (wings of the swan): The little finger of the *sarpa-sirsa* hand is stretched out.

Application: It represents the number 'six', construction of a bridge, accepting, rejecting, embrace (two hands), steps, a woman, a small child (two hand-palms facing), eyes, palm leaf for writing, hearing, blessing, saying 'come', the body.

25. *Samdamsa* (pincers): The fingers of the *padma-kosa* are brought close to one another and are drawn apart in quick succession.

Application: It denotes the belly, offering to deities, wound, great fear, worship, the number 'five'.

26. *Mukula* (flower bud): All the fingers are curved and brought together without touching.

Application: It is used to denote a water lily, taking food, holding a seal, the navel, five flower-tipped arrows of Kamdev—the God of Love.

27. *Tamra-cuda* (cock): The first finger of the *mukula* hand is separated and curved.

Application: It represents a cock, a crane, a cow, a camel, a pen, parrot, hook, noose, enmity (interlocked first fingers).

28. *Trishula* (trident): The thumb and the little finger are bent and joined, and the other three fingers are stretched and separated.

Application: It represents a *bel* (fruit) leaf, trident (weapon of Lord Shiva), the concept of trinity and the number 'three'.

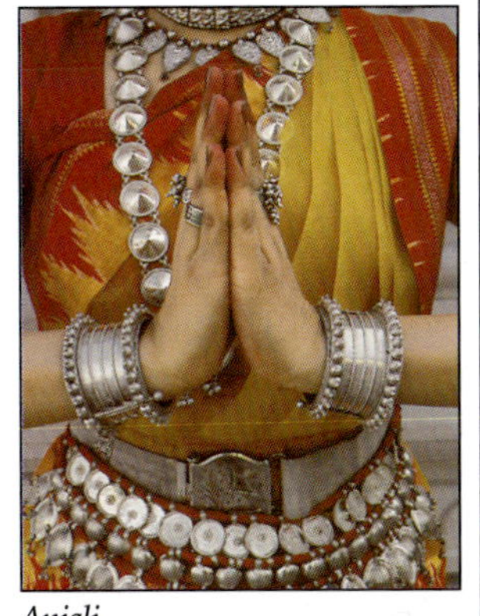

Anjali

Samyuta Hasta—Combined Hands

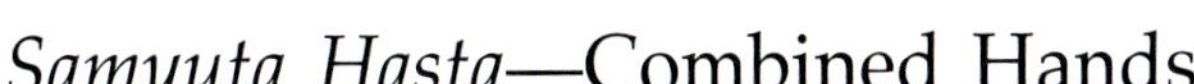

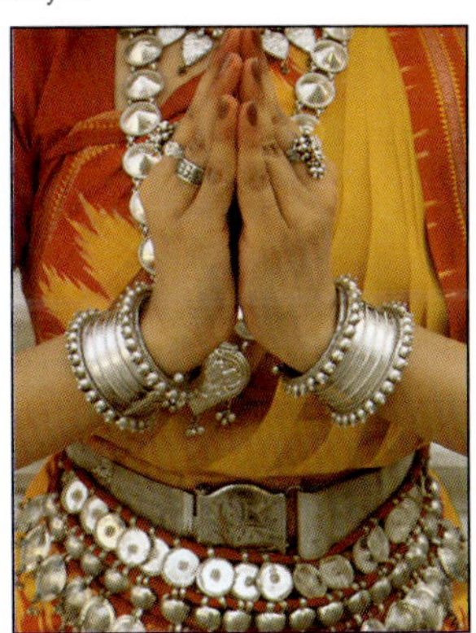

Kapota

1. *Anjali* (salutation): Two *pataka* hands join palms together in a gesture of salutation.

Application: It is held above the head to salute deities, before the face for preceptors and kings, and at the chest for equals.

2. *Kapota* (dove): Two *pataka* hands are joined at their base, sides and top with palms curved.

Application: It is used for salutation, addressing venerable persons, taking oath, acceptance and paying respect.

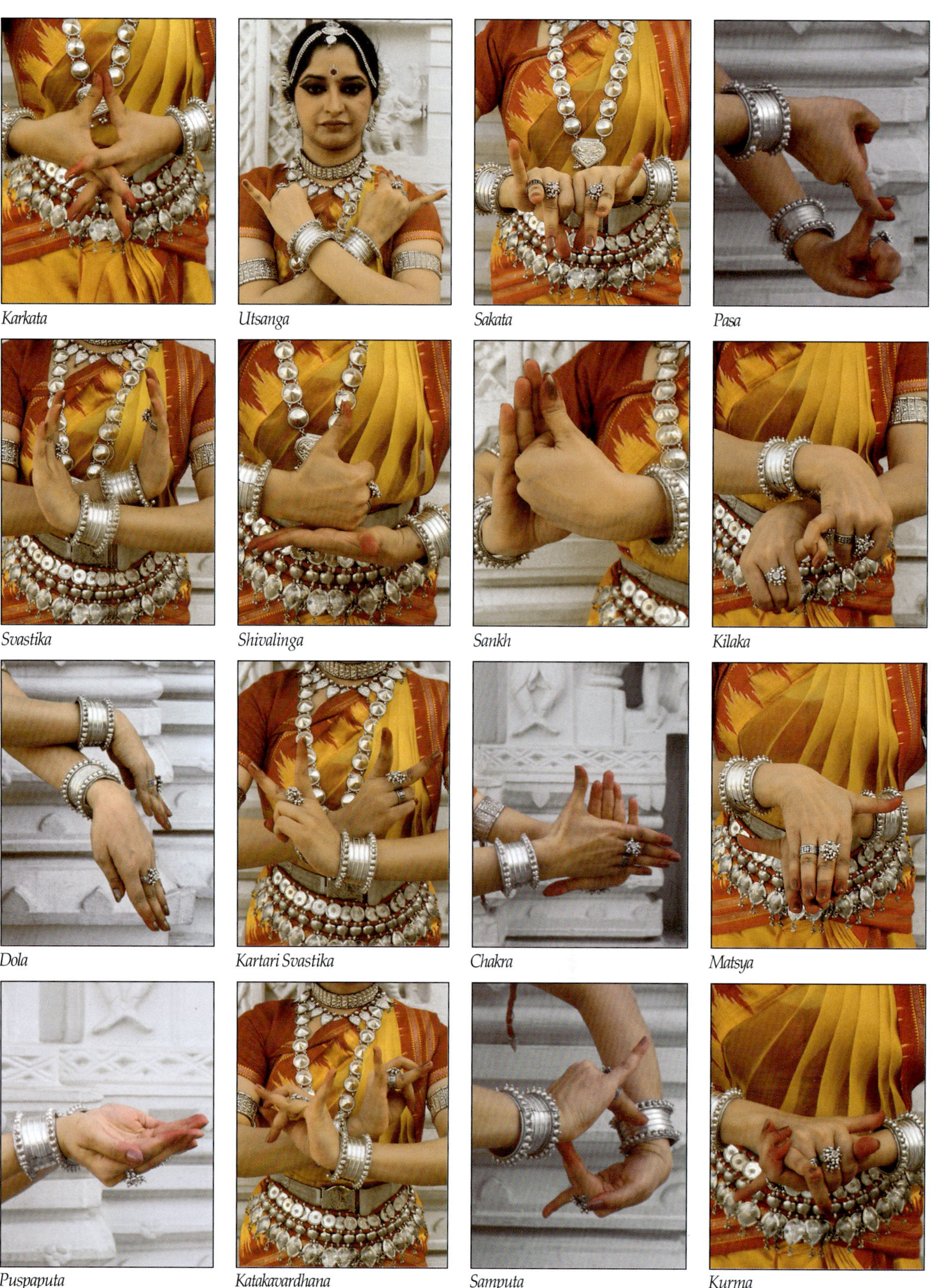
Karkata
Utsanga
Sakata
Pasa
Svastika
Shivalinga
Sankh
Kilaka
Dola
Kartari Svastika
Chakra
Matsya
Puspaputa
Katakavardhana
Samputa
Kurma

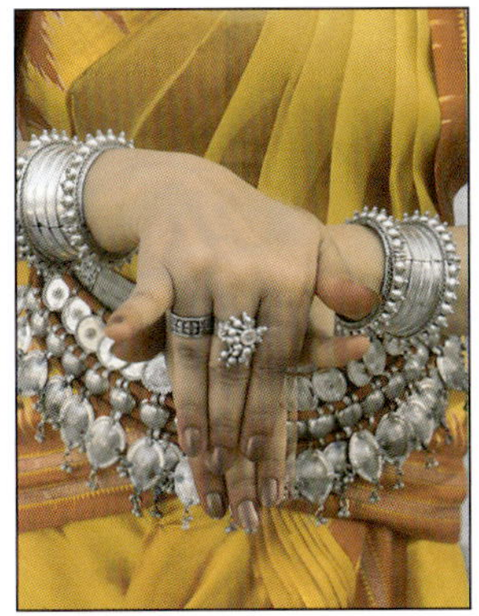
Varaha

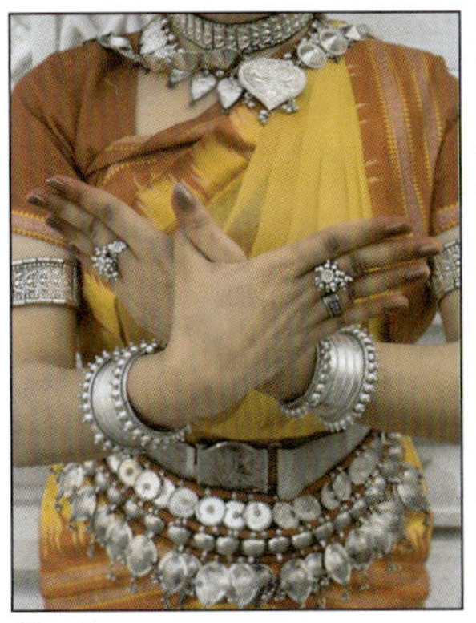
Garuda

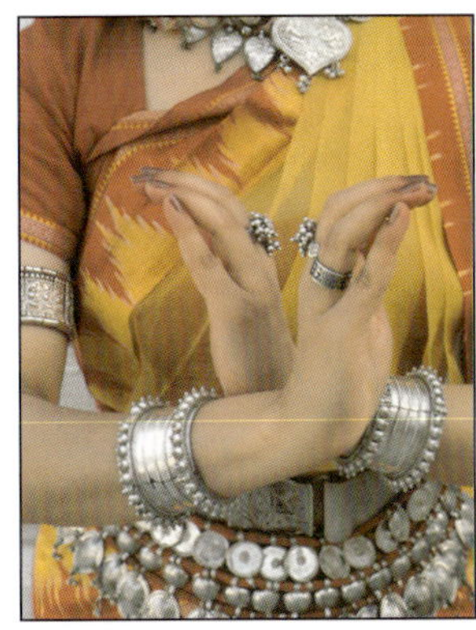
Naga-bandha

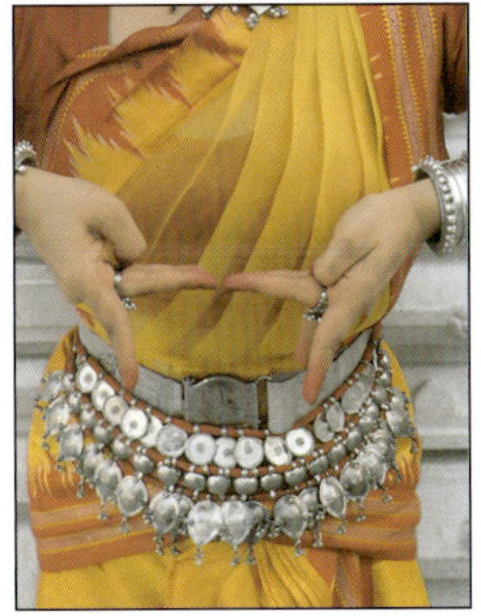
Khatva

3. *Karkata* (crab): The fingers of one hand are introduced into the spaces between fingers, with palms facing each other.

Application: It is used to express grief, anxiety, blowing a conch shell, bending the branch of a tree, coming together of a multitude, showing belly, stretching of limbs (arms overhead, palms turned upward).

4. *Svastika* (crossed): The two *tripataka* hands are crossed at the wrists and held vertically.

Application: It is used to represent crocodile, the gods (held above the head).

5. *Dola*: The *pataka* hands are held on the sides near the thighs.

Application: It is used at the beginning of the dance.

6. *Puspaputa* (flower basket): The *sarpa-sirsa* hands are joined along the sides, with palms up.

Application: It denotes waving lights (*arati*), receiving flowers, rice, fruits, water offering, drinking water, offering to gods.

7. *Utsanga* (embrace): The *mrga-sirsa* hands are crossed on the breast as in an embrace, with the fingertips touching shoulders.

Application: It is used to show an embrace, displaying armlets, shyness, instruction of children.

8. *Shivalinga* (Shiva's symbolic phallus): When the *ardha-chandra* is held by the left hand and the *sikhara* by the right hand, the *shivalinga* hand is formed.

Application: It denotes Shiva or *shivalinga.*

9. *Katakavardhana*: When a *svastika* is made by placing two *kataka-mukha* hands at the wrists the *katakavardhana* gesture is formed.

Application: An auspicious symbol used to depict, for instance, coronation, worship, marriage.

10. *Kartari Svastika* (crossed scissors): In this type of gesture, a *svastika* is made with the *kartari-mukha* hands crossed at the wrists.

Application: It is used to denote trees, branches, peaks of mountains (held high at the side).

11. *Sakata*: The middle finger of the *bhramara* hands is stretched.

Application: It is used in playing the role of a demon (*raksasa*).

12. *Sankh* (conch shell): The thumb of the *ardha-chandra* left hand is clasped by the fingers of the *musti* right hand with its thumb pressing the fingertips of the other hand.

Application: It denotes the conch shell symbol of Vishnu, blowing a conch.

13. Chakra (discus): The *ardha-chandra* hands are crossed with palms in contact.

Application: It denotes the discus symbol of Vishnu, a weapon (discus), a wheel.

14. Samputa (casket): In this type of gesture the fingers of the *chakra* hand are curved.

Application: It is used to denote concealing and covering things, casket, box.

15. Pasa (noose): The forefingers of the *suci* hands are interlocked and bent.

Application: It denotes enmity, a quarrel, noose, chain.

16. Kilaka (bond): The little fingers of the two *mrga-sirsa* hands are interlocked.

Application: It denotes affection, lovers' conversation.

17. Matsya (fish): The two *ardha-chandra* hands with palms down, the right hand on the back of the left hand, the thumbs are extended and move along with the rhythm.

Application: It denotes a fish, *matsya avatara*—the fish incarnation of Vishnu and the sea.

18. Kurma (tortoise): The fingers of the *chakra* hand are bent, except the thumb and little fingers, which are extended and move along with the rhythm.

Application: It denotes the *kurma avatara* of Vishnu, a tortoise.

19. Varaha (boar): The *mrga-sirsa* hands are placed one on the back of the other (palms down). The thumbs and little fingers are extended.

Application: It represents the *varaha avatara* of Vishnu.

20. Garuda (eagle mount): The *ardha-chandra* hands are held crossed with palms facing the body, and thumbs interlocked.

Application: It represents the symbol of *garuda*—the eagle mount of Lord Vishnu.

21. Naga-bandha (serpent tie): In this type of gesture the *sarpa-sirsa* hands are crossed (*svastika*).

Application: It is used to denote a pair of snakes, a bower (held high).

22. Khatva (bed): The fingertips of the two *chatura* hands are touced with forefingers and little fingers pointing down.

Application: It represents bed, litter.

23. Bherunda (birds): In this type of gesture the two *kapitta* hands are joined at the wrists.

Application: It denotes a pair of *bherunda* birds.

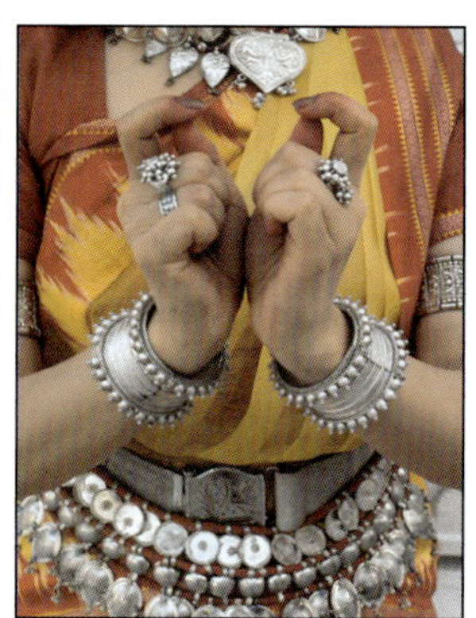

Bherunda

Following double spread: A young duo striking an Odissi bhangi *at the Udayagiri Khandagiri Caves.*

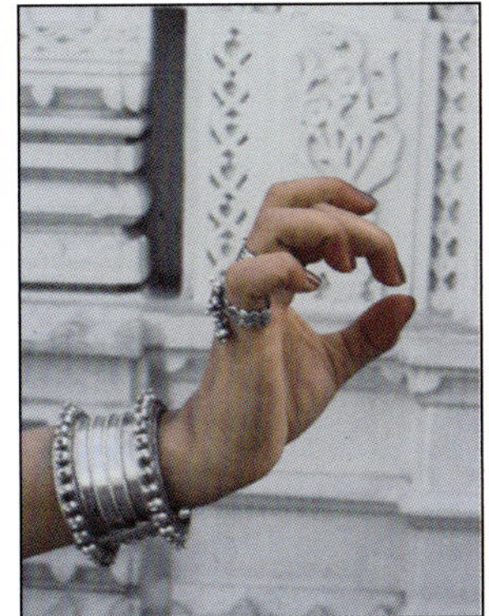
Shuk Chanchu

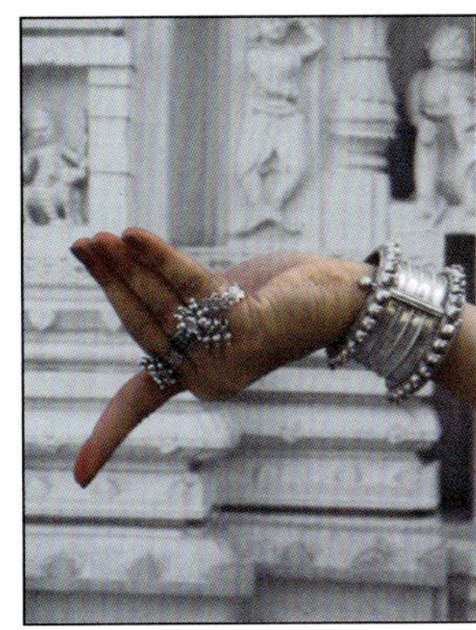
Prabhodhika

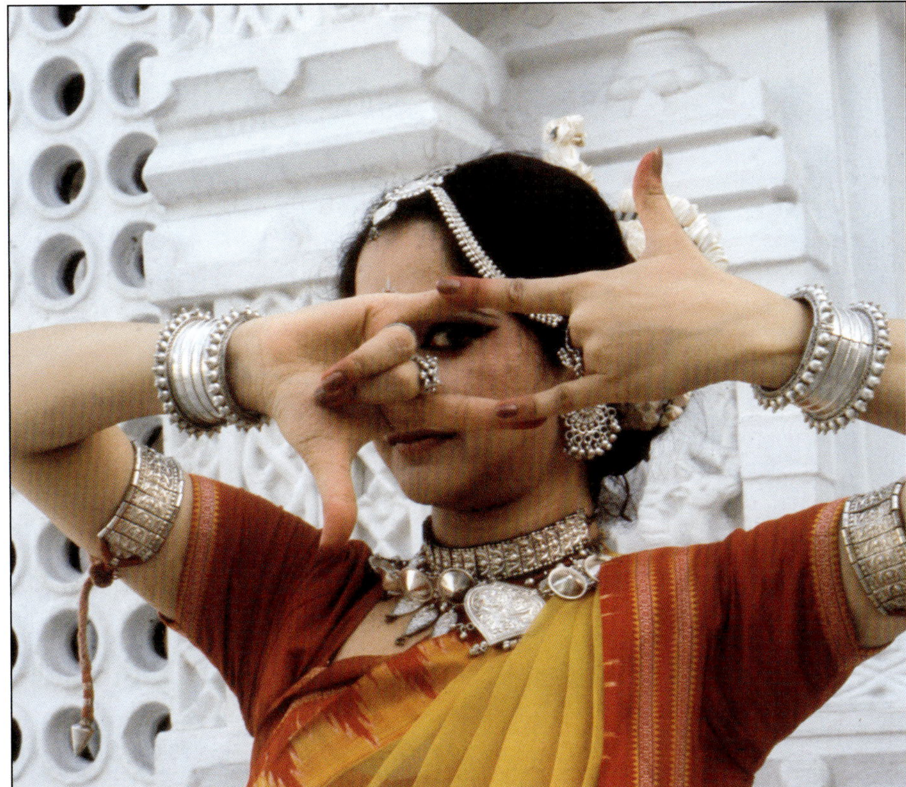
Gavaksha

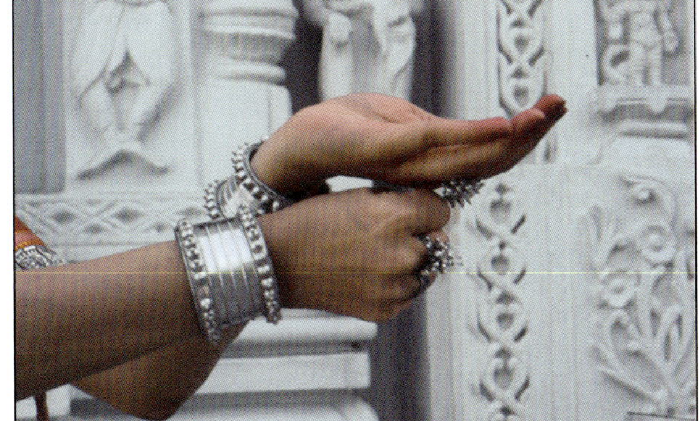
Pradeep

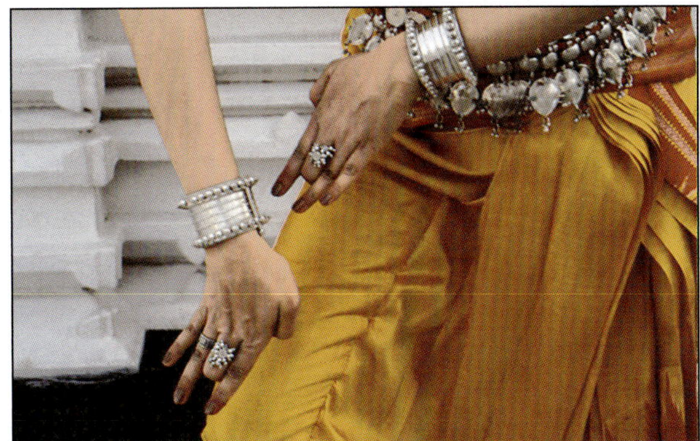
Vastra

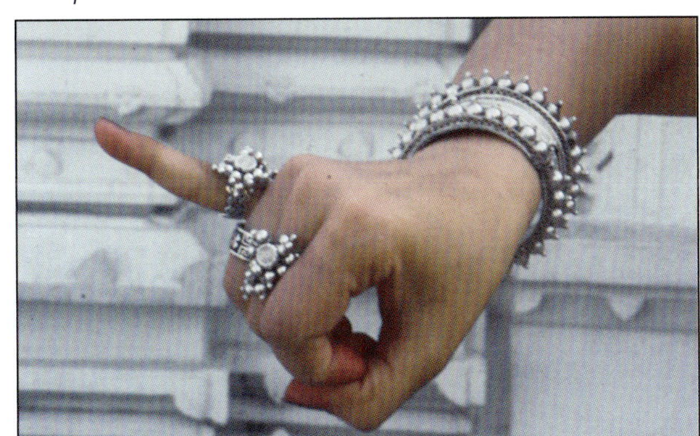
Bana

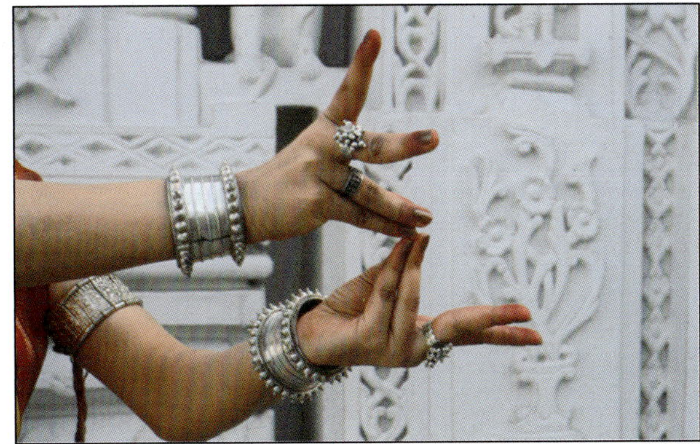
Ubhaya Kartari

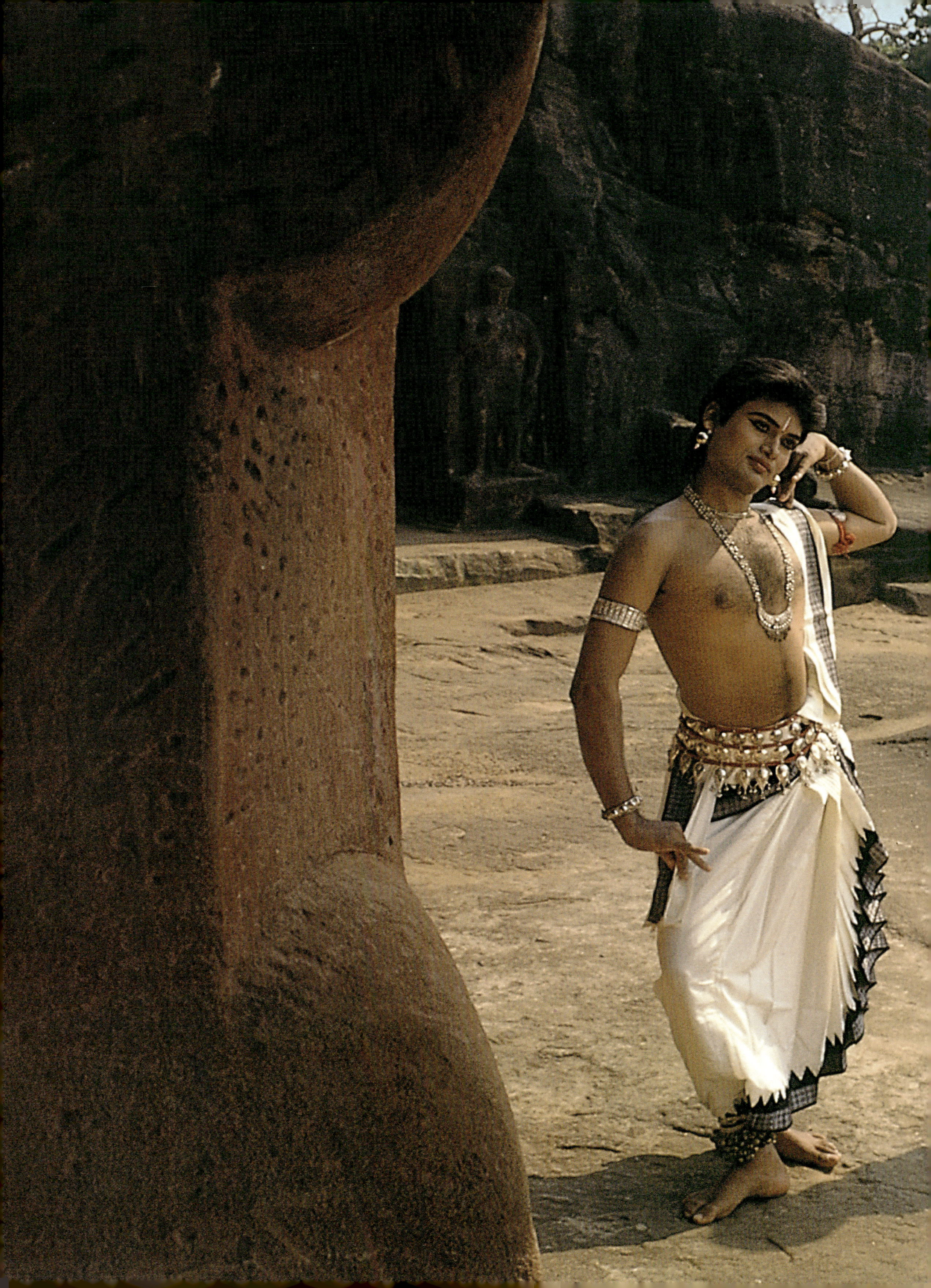

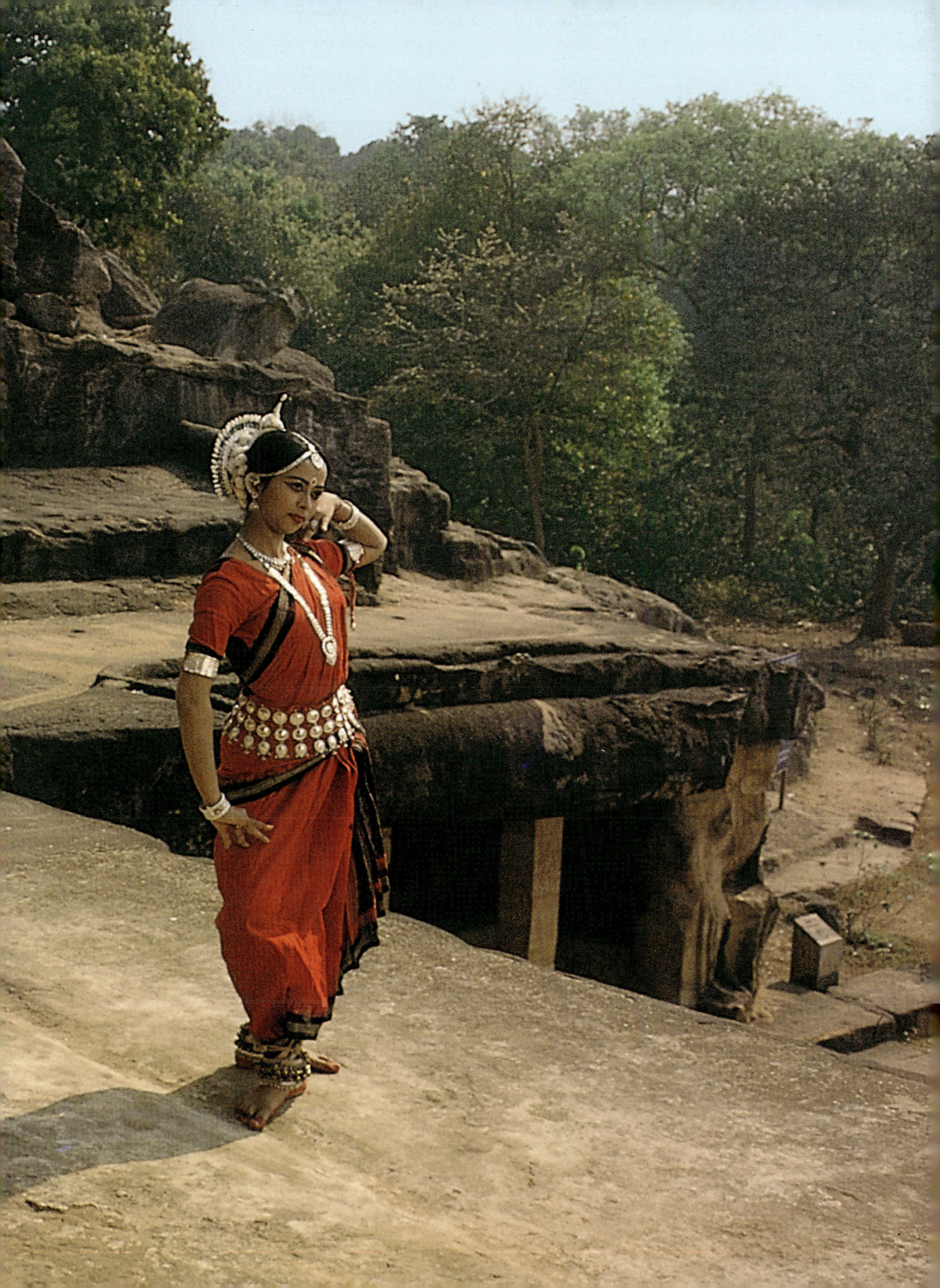

The *hastas* peculiar to Odissi, mentioned in the ancient Oriya scripture *Abhinaya Chandrika* are:

1. *Shuk Chanchu*	6. *Astra*	11. *Kadamba*
2. *Prabhodhika*	7. *Ubhaya Kartari*	12. *Nikunchaka*
3. *Gavaksha*	8. *Dhanu*	13. *Trisikha*
4. *Pradeep*	9. *Lulita*	14. *Chaturmukha*
5. *Bana*	10. *Tambula*	

Though Odissi strictly follows Nandikeswara's code in *Hasta,* it adheres to its own Oriya text also.

Repertoire of Odissi Dance

During the period of its rediscovery, the performance of Odissi consisted of one continuous piece of blended items, lasting about 15 to 20 minutes, which began with an invocation, *bhumipranam,* and lead into *batu, pallavi, abhinaya* and ended with *mokshya,* which was pure dance. Contemporary Odissi has undergone considerable change and expansion. One continuous piece of performance has been separated into distinct divisions and a repertoire created and expanded. In keeping with Odissi's devotional roots, most of the items are put into dance to express this devotional essence. The *bhava* is chaste and pure.

Mangalacharan

An invocatory piece, the auspicious beginning to any Odissi recital is the *mangalacharan.* The dancer enters the stage with stylised graceful movements and offers flowers or *pushpanjali* and performs *bhumipranam,* which is salutation to Mother Earth, by touching the ground with both the hands and then placing them on the forehead. This is followed by an invocation or *vandana,* which is in praise and worship of any god, such as Ganesha, Shiva, Rama, Krishna, Jagannath, Durga, Saraswati, and so on. The dancer expresses the *bhava* through *abhinaya* and *hastas.* After the invocation, the drummer plays the rhythmic syllables, which are traditionally fixed and are known as *ukutas.* The piece ends with *trikhandi pranam* (three-part salutation) in which the dancer pays salutation to gods, *gurus* and the audience.

Batu Nritya

This is a pure dance piece, in praise of Lord Shiva, depicting *Batuka Bhairav,* one of the 64 terrific aspects of Shiva. It begins with a series of sculpturesque poses representing body and hand movements, such as the playing of the *veena*, drum, flute and cymbals. Throughout the dance, the percussionist chants rhythmic syllables to the accompaniment of the percussion, but there is no song or recitation. Some *tala* variations are also introduced and each sequence of dance ends with a *tihai*. The dancer executes the variations in *tala* with her feet. The last sequence is always performed in the fast tempo.

Pallavi

Pallavi retains a special place in the Odissi recital. It is an item of pure dance that develops and grows as the variations in melody and rhythm are constantly expanded along with the movements. It begins with simple movements of pure dance and develops into complicated steps interwoven with rhythmic syllables. The grace, charm and fluid quality of this composition is punctuated by stylised poses from temple sculpture. It is the visual interpretation of the *raga*, which expands on notes, develops on rhythm and is enriched by intricate movements. The final result is harmony of music, dance and rhythm, which blossoms into a new creative identity. *Pallavi* can be seen as the step-by-step unfolding of petals into a beautiful flower. *Pallavis* are known by the *ragas* on which their music is based such as *saveri, kalyani, bajrakanti, shankaravarnam,* to name a few.

Abhinaya

One of the most challenging and important items of Odissi repertoire is *abhinaya*, or the expressive and interpretive dance. The dancer interprets emotions contained in a song or lyric with the support of *mukhabhinaya*, *hastabhinaya* and the *bhangis*. The dancer gives expression to the intensity of emotions through *bhava* contained in the lyrics.

The tradition of songs as we know it today in Orissa perhaps began in the 12th century with the well-known *ashtapadis* of Jayadeva. The Sanskrit songs of the *Geeta Govinda* are in direct ancestral line of songs and musical poetry in Orissa.

The romantic compositions of the *Geeta Govinda* are set in a slow tempo and the dancer gets complete flexibility to depict the emotion by gestures, glances and soft movements to convey clearly to the audience the richness and full meaning of the composition. In portraying the *bhava*, the dancer can bring out the myriad nuances of the *nayak-nayika* concept of Indian erotic literary legacy. Oriya songs also form the basis of *abhinaya* and are mostly compositions from the medieval Vaishnavite poets like Kavisurya Baldeva Ratha, Gopal Krishna Patnaik and Banamali Das. The love of Radha and Krishna is the all-time favourite theme for the poets.

Following double spread:
A nayika *lost in her thoughts when separated from her beloved.*

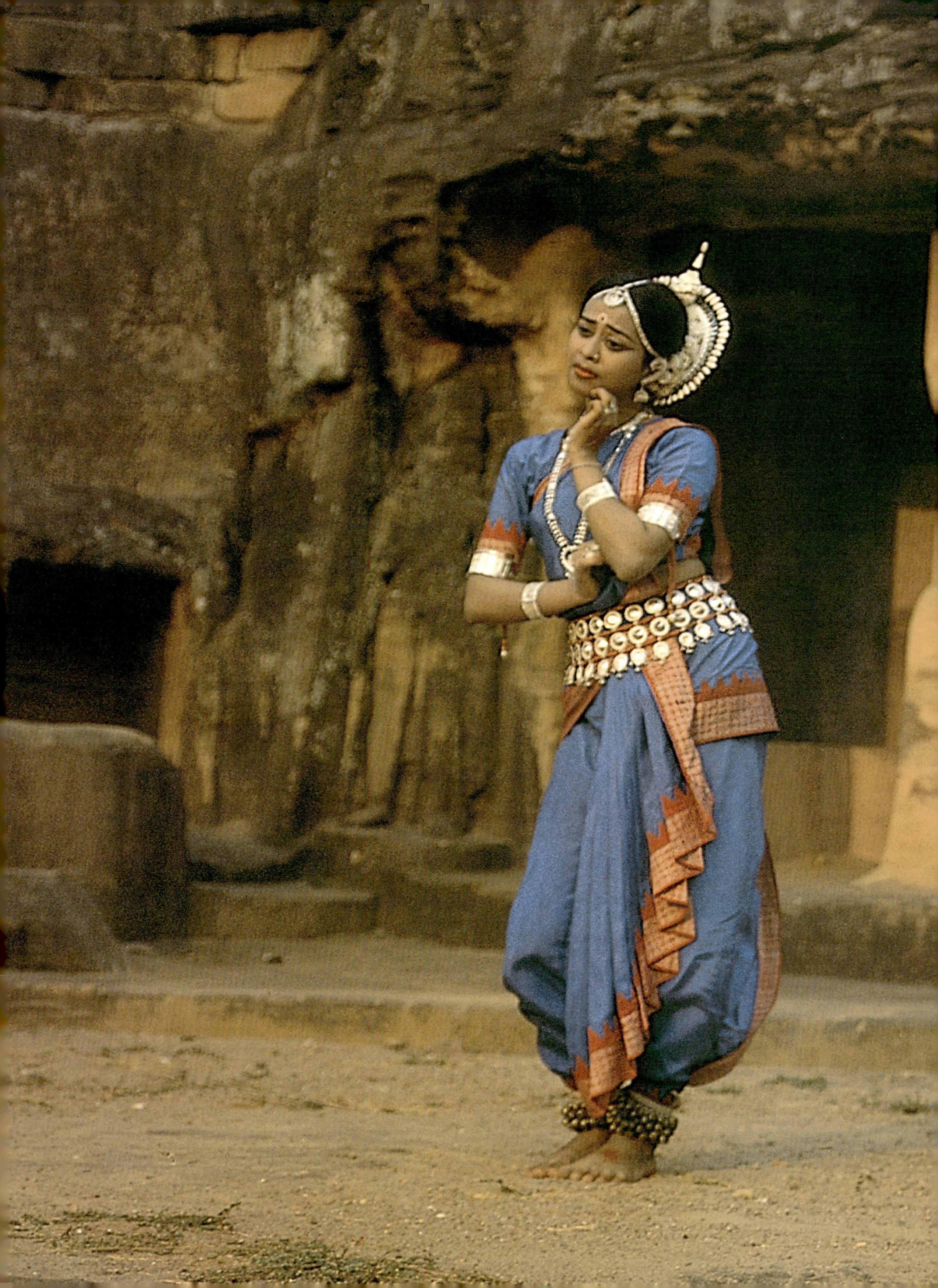

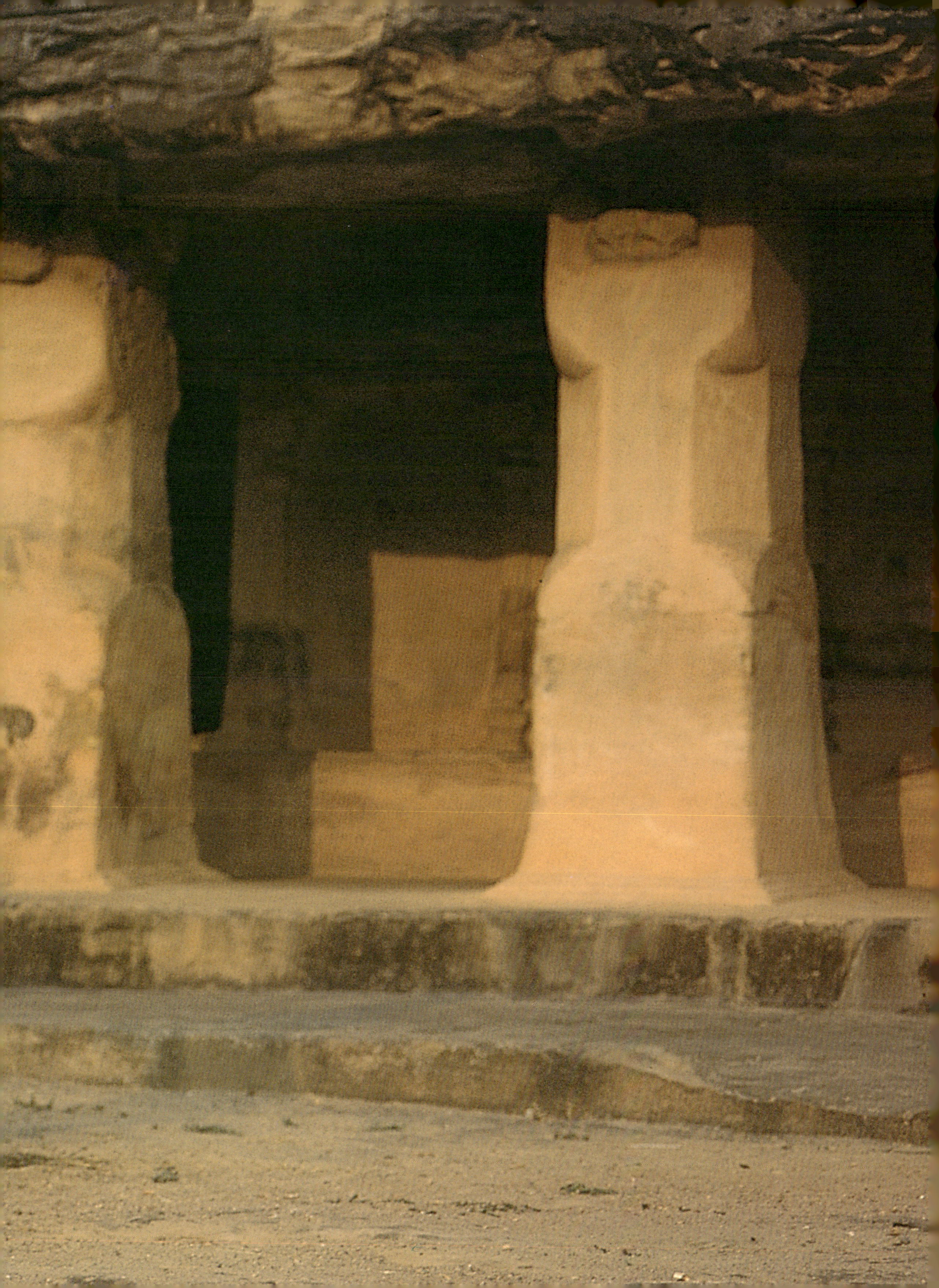

Moksha

Moksha is the concluding item of an Odissi recital. It is a pure dance composition. The tempo is fast and the dance builds to a crescendo accompanied by recitation and chanting of the rhythmic syllables, which are also played on the *mardala* (percussion instrument). It includes various patterns of *nritta,* but there is no music to accompany it except the rhythmic syllables. It is performed in a variety of *talas* like *pahapata, jhoola,* among others. 'In India, the ultimate aim of life is release (*moksha*) and art is one means of attaining this aim. *Moksha* is reintegration with the Absolute.' Thus in Odissi, the dance attuned to this ideal is known as *moksha naata*.

Note: A popular item of dance performed in the Sambalpur region of Orissa, *sabda swarpata,* was almost lost to the Odissi repertoire because during the years of restructuring of Odissi dance (1955-1956), it was not commonly performed. Of late this aspect has again attracted the attention of Odissi dance lovers who are trying to revive the lost glory of this beautiful aspect of Odissi tradition and pull it out of oblivion.

Music

Odissi has its own distinct system of music which is sweet, melodious and classical. The language of the songs is Sanskrit or Oriya. It is the only classical dance where the dance and music go by the same name, Odissi. Unrivalled in Odissi's musical repertoire is Jayadeva's *Geeta Govinda* and various songs of Oriya language. The *ashtapadis* are unique compositions in Sanskrit, and Jayadeva had specified *ragas* and *talas* for each. This tradition was well established by the 12th century. Other important texts were written on music in the 15th and 18th centuries. The Radha Krishna theme of the *Geeta Govinda* is expressed in very many poems in Oriya language, and these are sung and form part of the music of modern Odissi.

Traditional instruments used are percussion instruments known as the *pakhawaj* (in Oriya *mardala*), *gini* (a pair of small cymbals), *veena* and flute. Nowadays, the violin and *sitar* are also used.

Aharya: Costumes, Ornaments and Make-up of an Odissi Dancer

All four forms of *abhinaya* in the *Natya Shastra,* namely, *angika, vachika, sattvik* and *aharya,* are given due emphasis in Odissi. The last of these, *aharya*, relates to costume, ornamentation and make-up.

The *Abhinaya Chandrika* describes the costume to be worn by the Odissi dancer and also gives an elaborate description of ornaments and make-up.

Born out of the tradition of the *mahari,* who was considered a bride of Lord Jagannath, the contemporary classical Odissi dancer is also made-up and dressed like a bride. Although influenced by the mode of dress of the *maharis,* the costume of the contemporary dancer is specific to the modern version of Odissi and has a unique style of its own.

The Odissi dancer usually wears a bright coloured sari of indigenous silk, called *patta*. This is now tailored to allow greater freedom of movement and is akin to that worn by the *gotipuas*. The blouse, known as a *kancula,* was traditionally tight fitting, brightly coloured and decorated with imitation stones. The blouse worn today is a regular sari blouse. To cover the hips, an apron with frills, called a *nibibandha,* is worn, which is tied in the front. At the waist is tied a cord with tassels at both ends, called a *jhoba*.

The *Abhinaya Chandrika* contains an exhaustive list of ornaments for the entire body to be worn by the dancer and most of them can be seen represented in the temple sculptures of Orissa. These, however, are too numerous for practical purposes and the current trend is to use considerably fewer ornaments, which allows the dancer greater freedom of movement. An *alaka* is now usually the only ornament for the head, *kapa* for the ears, *chapasari* and *padakatilaka* for the neck, *tayita* for the arms, *karakankan* for the wrists. For the waist is *bengapatia,* which literary means frog's mouth, as the last row of this ornate waistband is made up of stylised frogs. All ornaments for the feet have been done away with except *nupura* on the ankles.

A crown of *shola* flowers is worn on the head embellished in the centre by *taya,* a tapering column of flowers. Earlier, make-up consisted of sandalwood paste or *chandan,* applied in the pattern of a creeper—*gorachana,* on the forehead above the eyebrows and down to the cheeks but, in contemporary times, white dots form this pattern. A *bindi* or spot of vermilion is applied in the centre of the eyebrows, a beauty spot on the chin and the eyes are highlighted with *kohl*. *Alata,* a red liquid, is applied on the palms of the hands.

Different styles of dressing the hair are mentioned in the *Abhinaya Chandrika,* but the contemporary dancer usually makes a bun or *puspachuda*—a hair-knot which is decorated with *shola* flowers.

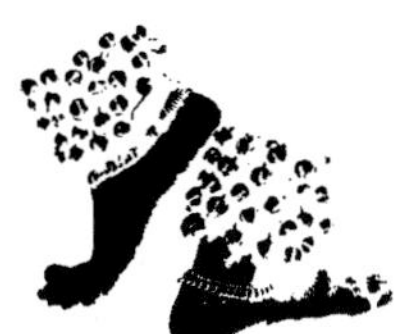

Following double spread: Odissi dancers in a group choreography depicting a sequence from the Mahabharata.

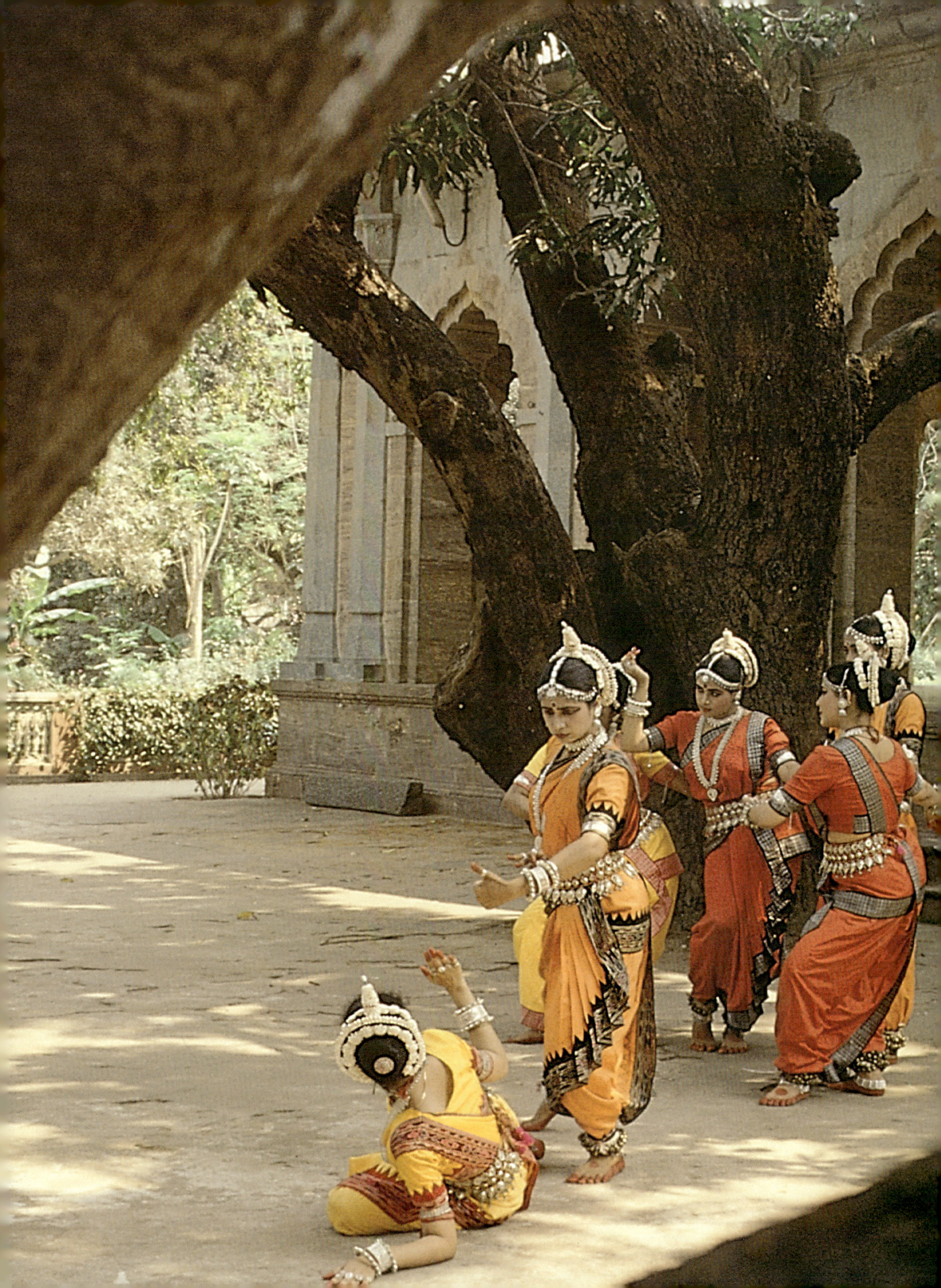

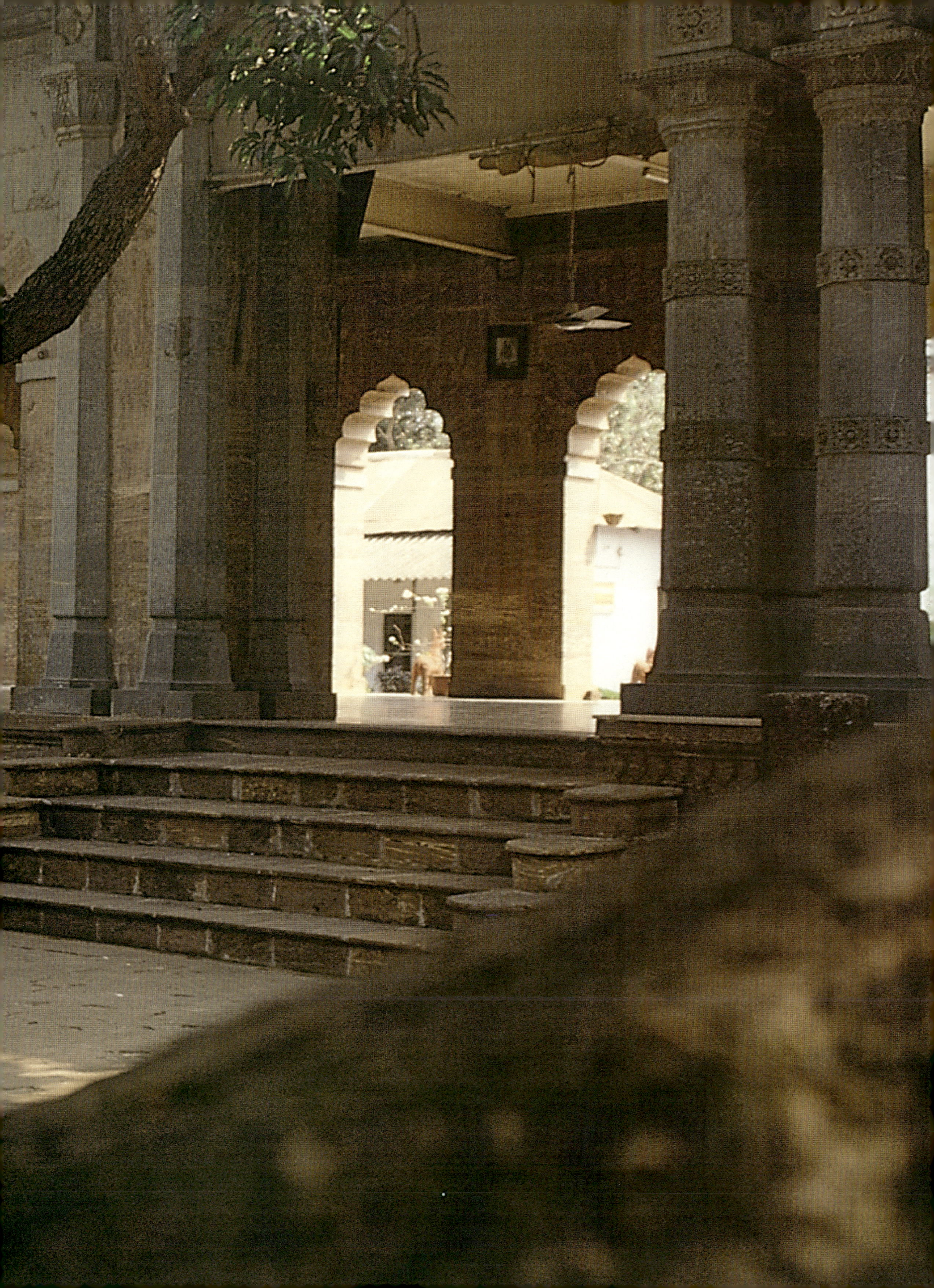

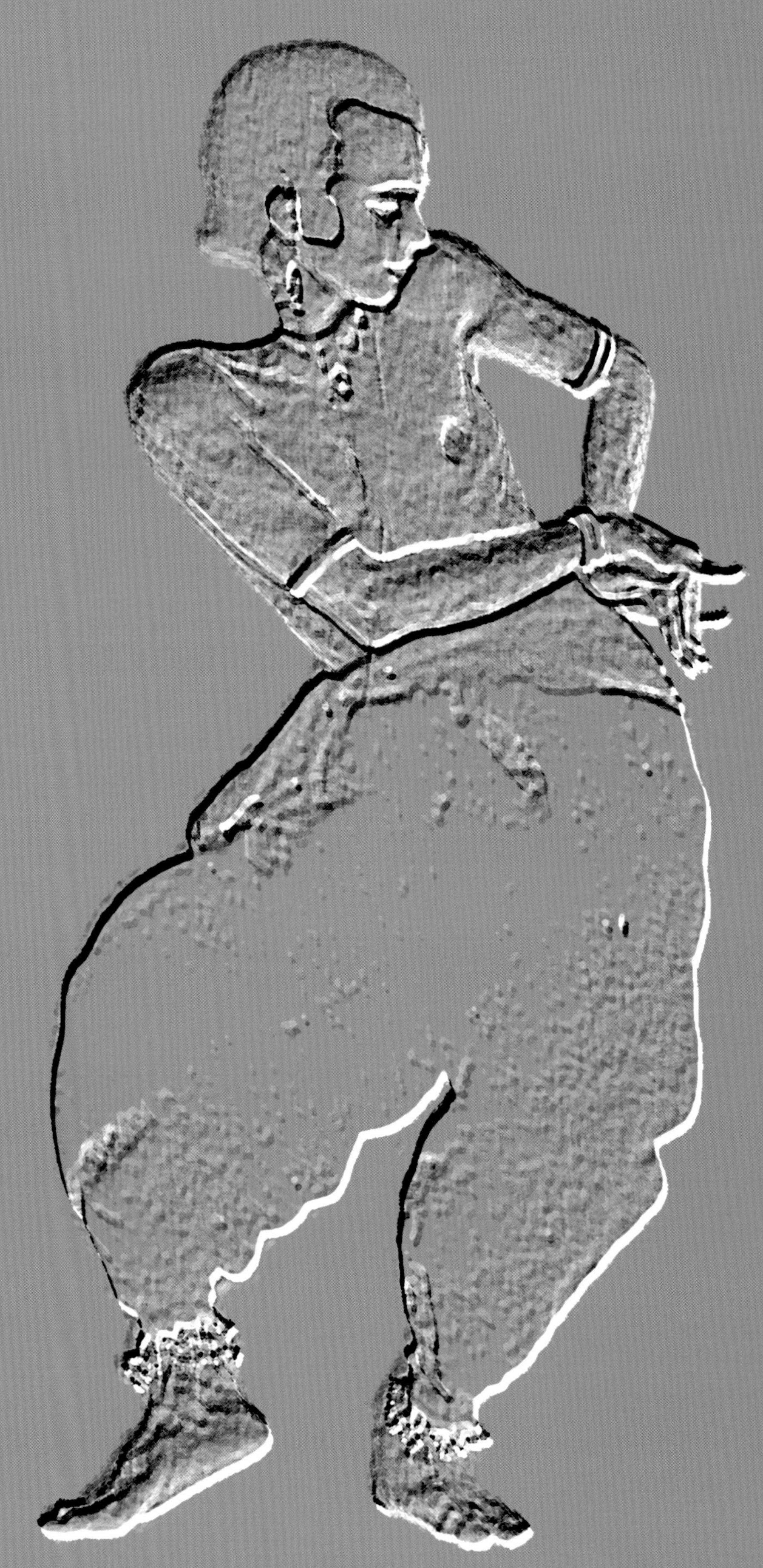

THE ARCHITECTS AND THE GURUS

Architects

Guru Pankaj Charan Das

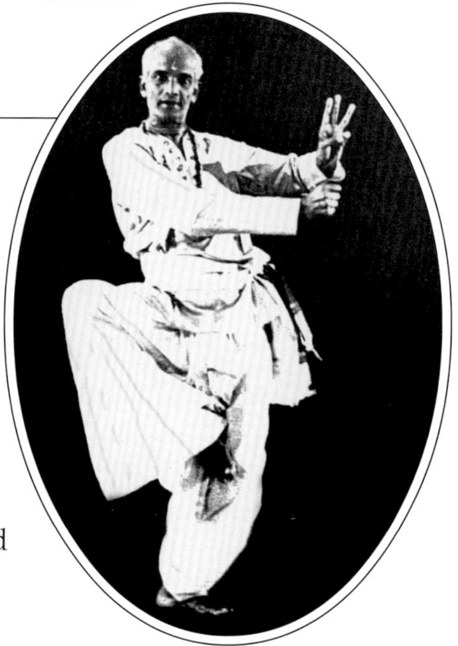

PURI

Guru Pankaj Charan Das was born in 1925 in the family of a *mahari*. He received his initial training in dance from his aunt Ratnaprabha *mahari*, and later from leading *gurus* of the *Raslila* groups, Ranganath Dev Goswami and Bhikari Charan Dalai. He was also trained as a *gotipua* dancer.

Widely respected as the guru of Odissi dance, he had guided and trained a number of dance teachers and dancers in his lifetime, including such eminent masters as Guru Kelucharan Mohapatra, Guru Mayadhar Raut, Guru Deba Prasad Das, Yamini Krishnamurty and Priyambada Mohanty. This earned him the affectionate title 'the *guru* of *gurus*'.

Guru Kelucharan Mohapatra

BHUBANESWAR

Guru Kelucharan Mohapatra made such immense contributions to Odissi dance as a teacher, performer, choreographer, researcher and system-builder that one identifies the last 50 years as the 'Kelucharan era of Odissi'. Born in Raghurajpur near Puri in a family of *patachitra* painters, as a child, he was trained as a *gotipua* and later joined the *Raslila* group, Annapurna Theatre, and distinguished himself as a dancer, percussionist and choreographer. In the later years, his choreography began to acquire the stunning beauty of sculptures in motion. His *abhinaya,* deep and imaginative, his playing the *pakhawaj* or *mardala* lend an extra dimension to his dance performances.

He trained innumerable outstanding dancers and teachers including Sanjukta Panigrahi, Sonal Mansingh, Madhvi Mudgal and Kumkum Mohanty.

He was honoured with various awards and felicitations, including the Padma Vibhushan, for his contribution and dedication to Odissi music. He ran a dance institute 'Srjan' in Bhubaneswar training talented students.

Guru Deba Prasad Das

BHUBANESWAR

Guru Deba Prasad Das was trained in Odissi dance by Mohan Chandra Mohapatra as a *gotipua*. Later he joined a theatre group as dance director. He shot into prominence when Indrani Rehaman took him along with her in various dance festivals. He played a prominent role in the movement for reviving Odissi dance. He was a gifted guru and had contributed significantly by his lyrical style and earthy flavour of *abhinaya*. He was the recipient of the Sangeet Natak Akademi Award and senior fellowship and trained many outstanding artistes.

Guru Mayadhar Raut

DELHI

Guru Mayadhar Raut was trained as a child in the art of *gotipua* dancing by his elder brother Harihar Raut. He joined many theatre companies like the other *gurus* and later joined Kala Vikash Kendra as a *guru* in 1952. He went to Kalakshetra College of Fine Arts, Madras and studied Bharatanatyam under Rukmuni Devi Arundale and acquired knowledge of the *Natya Shastra*. He choreographed several new dance pieces significantly enriching the Odissi repertoire. His style is distinct with fluidity and grace. He has been resident *guru* at the Sri Ram Bhartiya Kala Kendra in Delhi and has trained several accomplished dancers like Aloka Paniker, Kiran Segal, Geeta Mahalik and Ranjana Gauhar, the author of the present volume. For his contribution, he has received many awards including the Sangeet Natak Akademi Award.

Gurus

Guru Hare Krishna Behera

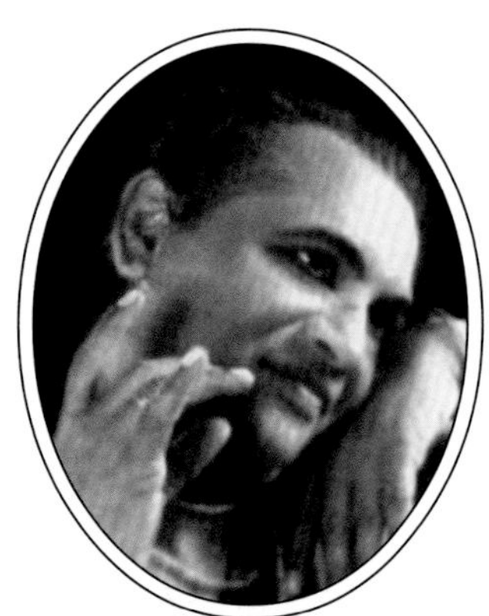

DELHI

Guru Hare Krishna Behera's artistic journey began when, at the age of six, he was admitted to the village *jatra* party. He was recognised by his first guru, Ramhari Behera, from whom he learnt both *gotipua* and present-day Odissi. Then he started learning from Shri Ram Chandra Dey, Shri Ramchandra Mahapatra and Guru Kelucharan Mohapatra. He founded the Guru Hare Krishna Behera College of Art and Culture and Bhartiya Nritya Sangeet Kala Parishad in his native town, Balasore. He was awarded the prestigious Sangeet Kala Akademi Award.

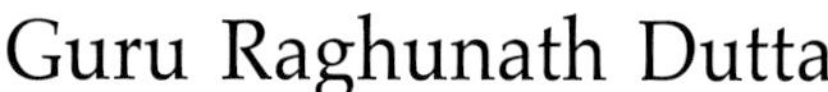

Guru Raghunath Dutta

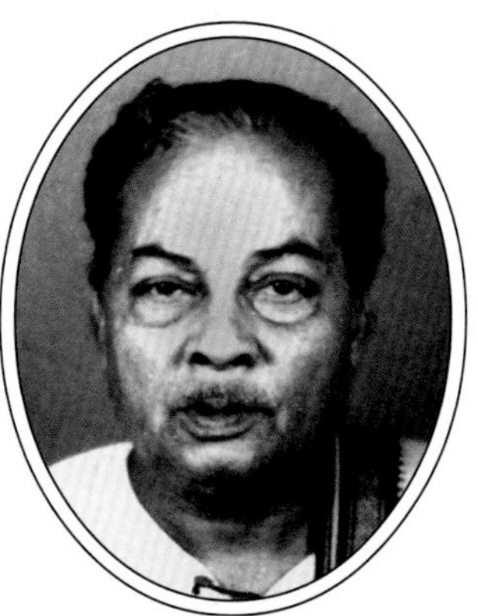

CUTTACK

Shri Raghunath Dutta prepared for a career as a dance teacher by assisting Guru Kelucharan Mohapatra in his training work. He has trained a large number of dancers and has enriched the Odissi dance repertoire through his compositions. He has received the Sangeet Natak Akademi Awards, both Central and State.

Guru Gangadhar Pardhan

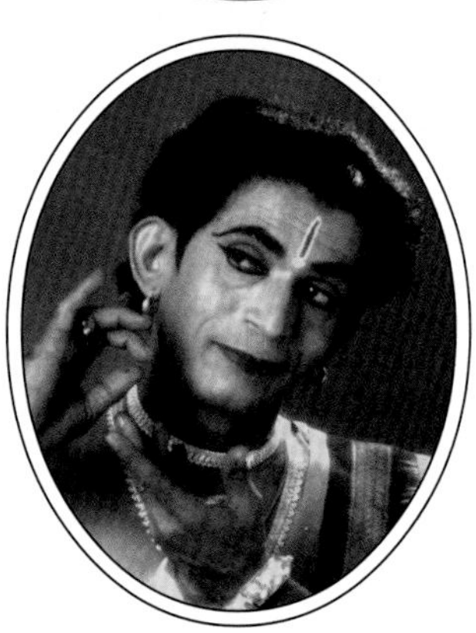

BHUBANESWAR

Guru Gangadhar Pardhan was initiated into the *gotipua* dance tradition from the age of six. He completed his Natyacharya course in Odissi dance from the Utkal Sangeet Mahavidyalay and was further trained under Late Guru Pankaj Charan Das, Late Guru Deba Prasad Das, Dr Minati Mishra and Shri Dhirendra Nath Patnaik.

He received intensive training in *mardala* under the tutelage of the legendary master Late Singhari Shyama Sundar Kar and Guru Banmali Maharana. He established the Orissa Dance Academy in 1975 at Bhubaneswar and subsequently opened its branches in both India and abroad.

He also set up the Konark Natya Mandap in the year 1985, where the Konark Dance and Music Festival is held. He has equally excelled as choreographer, composer, director, dance *guru* and organiser of festivals, and was honoured with the Sangeet Natak Akademi Awards, both Central and State.

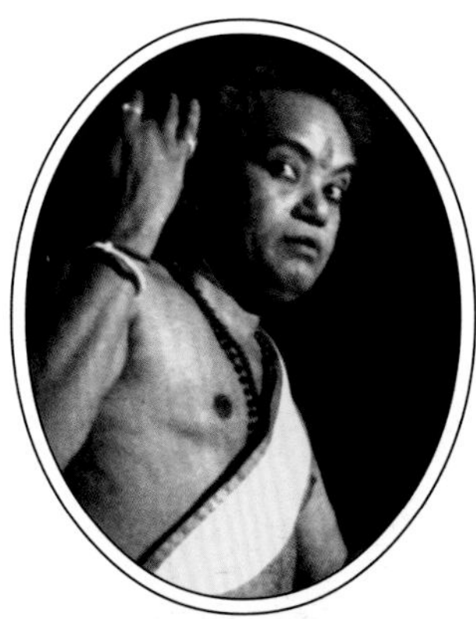

Guru Ramani Ranjan Jena

CUTTACK

Guru Ramani Ranjan Jena has received the Orissa Sangeet Natak Akademi Award and is known both as a teacher and performer. He received his Master's degree, from Kala Vikash Kendra. He taught at Kalakshetra College of Fine Arts, Madras, and later set up his own school called Kamala Kala Pitha in Cuttack.

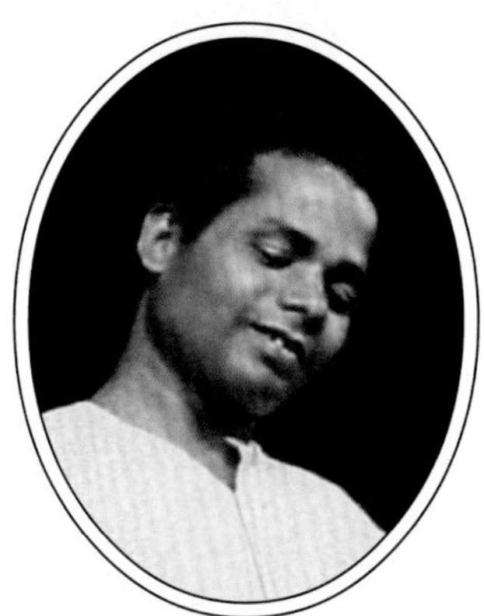

Guru Durga Charan Ranbir

BHUBANESWAR

Guru Durga Charan Ranbir is a senior disciple of Guru Deba Prasad Das and a renowned teacher of Odissi dance. He has established himself as the most prominent representative of the Deba Prasad school of Odissi dance and has made notable contribution with several choreographic creations of his own. He has trained a large number of well-known dancers and has travelled widely, presenting his disciples in national and international festivals, and has set up his own institution 'Nrityayan'. He has been awarded senior fellowship and the Orissa Sangeet Natak Akdemi Award.

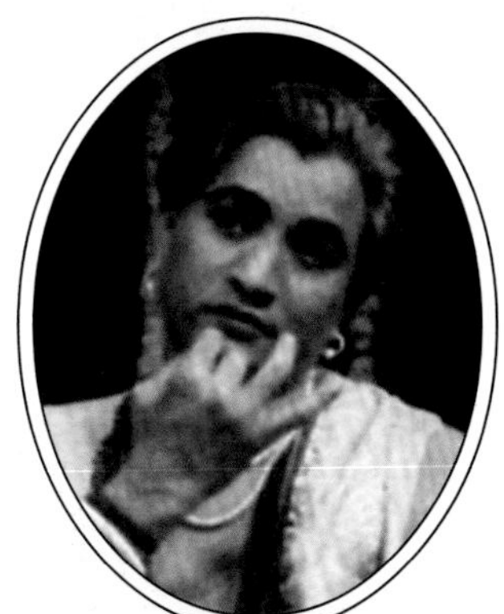

Guru Natabar Maharana

MUMBAI

Guru Natabar Maharana was trained in Odissi by many *gurus* but mainly by Guru Kelucharan Mohapatra. He runs his own institute in Mumbai and is well-versed in the playing of *pakhawaj*. He has trained many well-known dancers.

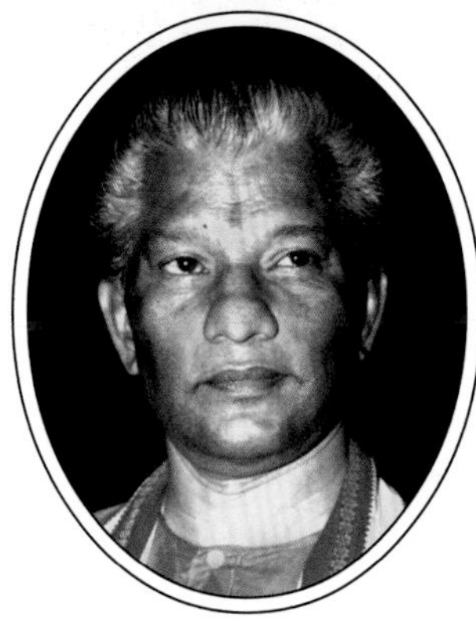

Guru Trinath Maharana

DELHI

Guru Trinath Maharana began studying as a *gotipua* at a very early age. He started his Odissi training with Guru Pankaj Charan Das and later with Guru Kelucharan Mohapatra. He taught in various schools in Orissa before settling down in Delhi. He is a proficient *pakhawaj* player and has choreographed dance dramas and group compositions. He trains many young dancers at his institution in Delhi.

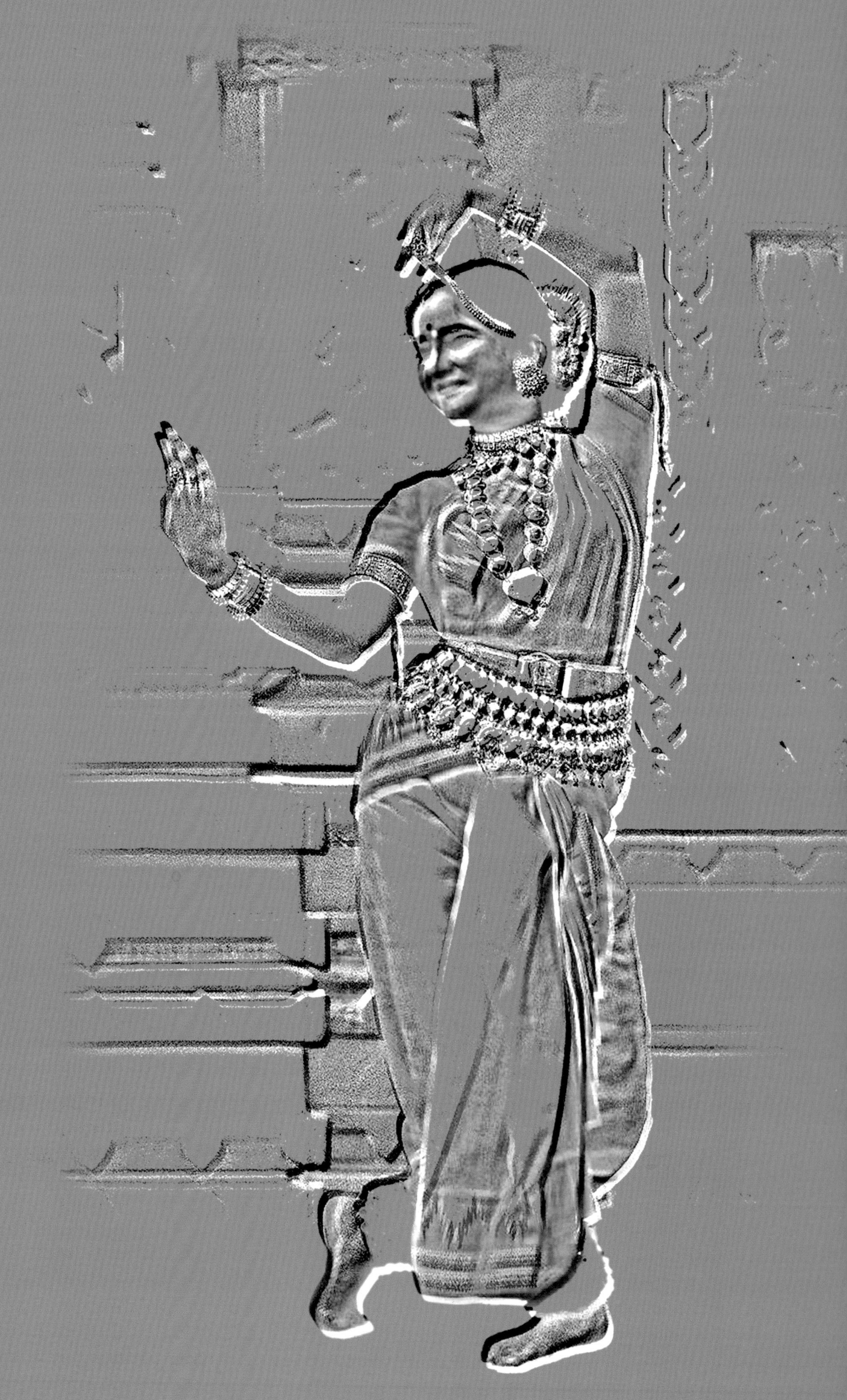

DANCERS—Vehicles of Expression

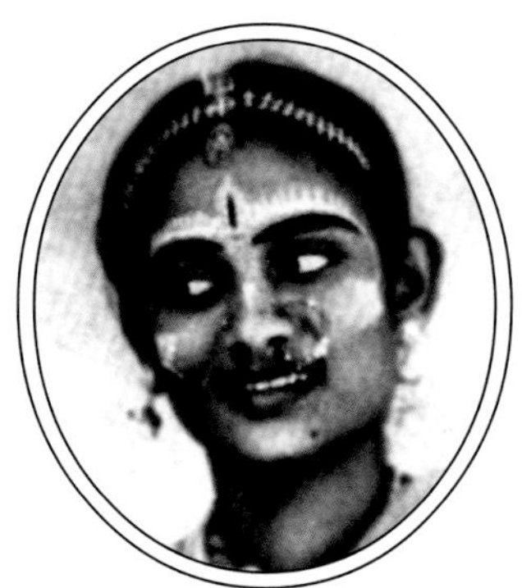

Priyambada Mohanty

BHUBANESWAR

Priyambada Mohanty was trained in Odissi dance by Guru Pankaj Charan Das, Guru Kelucharan Mohapatra and Guru Deba Prasad Das. She happens to be the dancer whose performances at the Youth Festival in Delhi in 1954 helped Odissi gain recognition as a classical dance art. A scholar by profession, she has also served as the chairperson of Orissa Sangeet Natak Akademi.

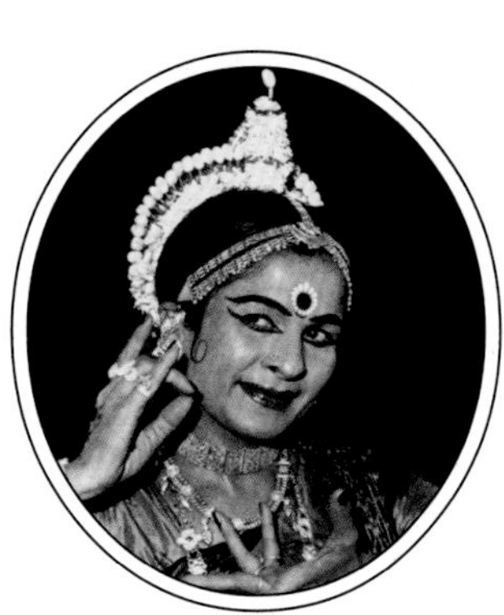

Sanjukta Panigrahi

BHUBANESWAR

A pioneer of Odissi dance, Sanjukta Panigrahi started her training with Guru Kelucharan Mohapatra at a very young age. She rendered valuable service to Odissi by taking it to all parts of the world. Her name is synonymous with Odissi. Her performances reflected an intense inner vitality and poise, lending her dance a quality which sets her apart from her contemporaries. Sanjukta received several honours, like the Padma Shree and Sangeet Natak Akademi Awards, which she shared with her husband Raghunath Panigrahi for their services to Odissi.

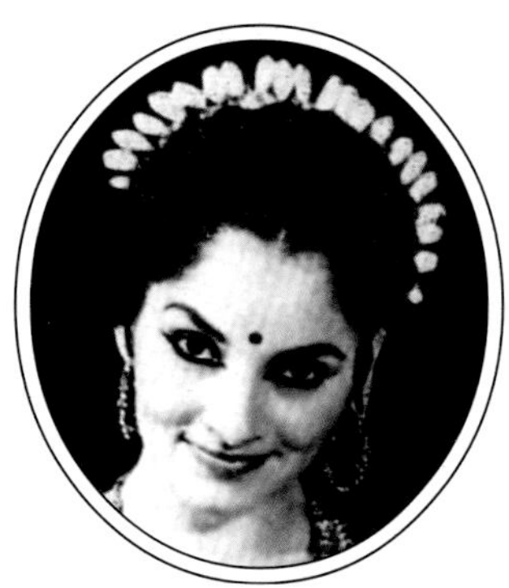

Indrani Rehman

DELHI

Indrani Rehman was already an established Bharatnatyam dancer when she took to Odissi training under Guru Deba Prasad Das. To her goes the credit for bringing Odissi to the national and international platform by performing it extensively. With her attractive stage presence and refined taste, she contributed substantially to the development of Odissi as a major classical dance form.

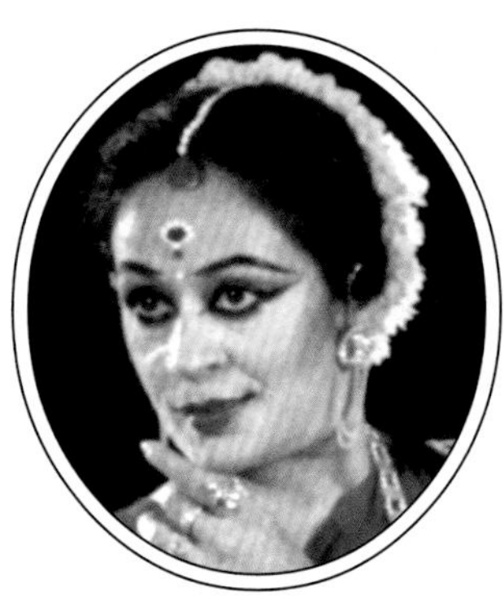

Sonal Mansingh

DELHI

A renowned personality of Indian dance and recipient of the Padma Vibhusan, Sonal Mansingh was trained in both Odissi and Bharatnatyam. She is known for her innovative interpretation of traditional themes as also for her choreographic works marked by contemporary sensitivity. She has performed extensively at home and abroad. She founded the Centre for Indian Classical Dances (CICD) in Delhi and has trained many young dancers. Sonal Mansingh is today the acknowledged master of interpreting India through dance and related artistic traditions.

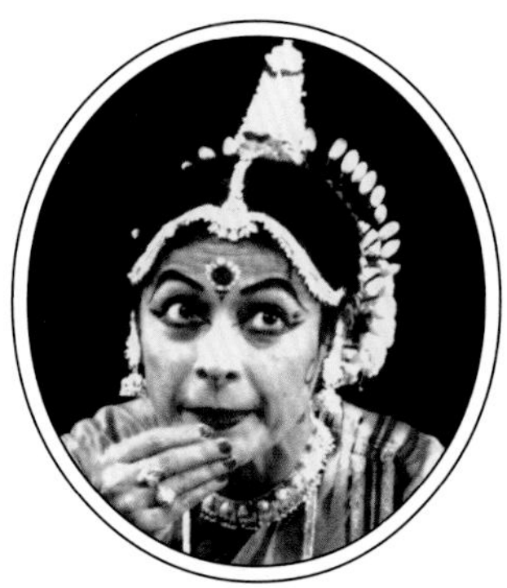

Kumkum Mohanty

BHUBANESWAR

Kumkum Mohanty started Odissi at the age of nine in Kala Vikas Kendra, Cuttack. She is inextricably linked with the evolution of modern Odissi dance. One of the leading disciples of Guru Kelucharan Mohapatra, she has performed all over the country. At present, she heads the Odissi Reasearch Centre for promoting and propagating the Odissi dance form and Odissi music.

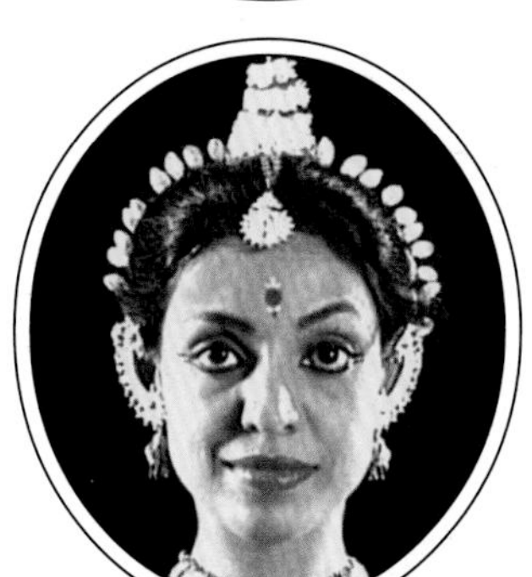

Madhvi Mudgal

DELHI

Madhvi Mudgal is the premier disciple of Guru Kelucharan Mohapatra. A leading performer of Odissi style, she has contributed substantially to Indian dance by choreographing group productions. She is an outstanding teacher and has been honoured with several awards—Sanskriti, Padma Shree, and Sangeet Natak Akademi Award.

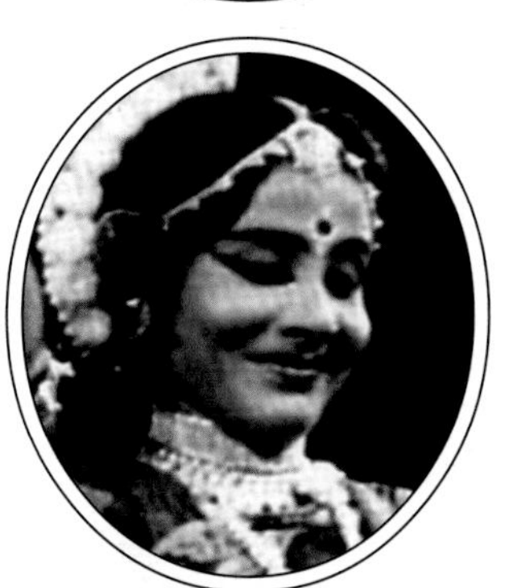

Aloka Paniker

DELHI

Aloka Paniker trained under Guru Mayadhar Raut in Odissi dance at the Bharatiya Kala Kendra. She later joined it as a teacher. Aloka hails from a family of stage and screen artistes and has won critical acclaim for her solo performances in India and abroad.

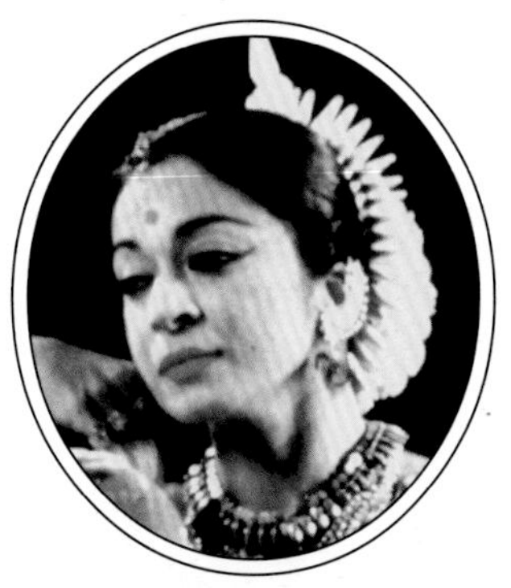

Kiran Segal

DELHI

Kiran Segal is a senior diciple of Guru Mayadhar Raut and is a leading exponent of Odissi style. She has performed extensively and is also a dedicated teacher. She has enriched the Odissi style with several of her own compositions and choreographic works. She has been honoured with the Padma Shree and Sangeet Natak Akademi Awards.

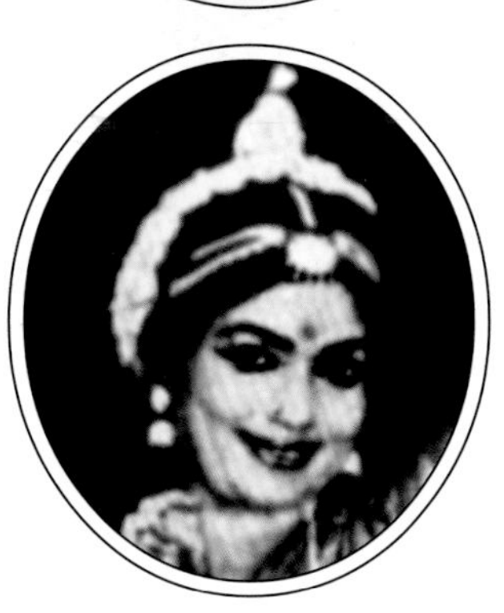

Minati Mishra

BHUBANESWAR

Minati Mishra is a senior acclaimed dancer who trained in Odissi dance under Guru Kelucharan Mohapatra and Guru Deba Prasad Das. She has received the Sangeet Natak Akademi Awards, both Central and State.

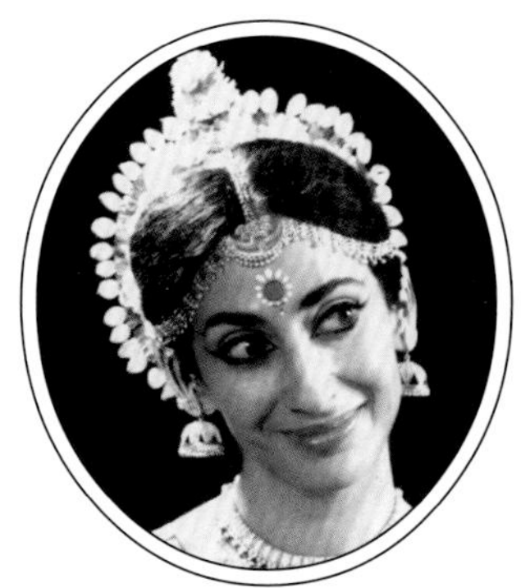

Sharon Lowen

DELHI

Sharon Lowen, an American-born Odissi dancer, trained under Guru Kelucharan Mohapatra. She has written scholarly articles on Indian dance traditions and has won the Sahitya Kala Parisad Samman. Besides performances in India and abroad, she has scripted, produced and choreographed for theatre, film and television.

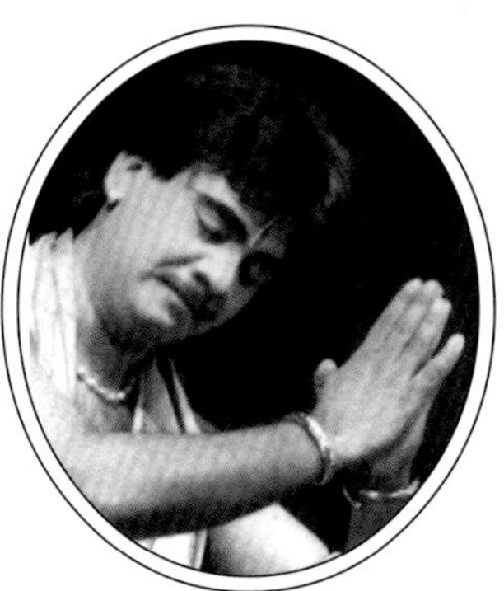

Ratikanta Mohapatra

BHUBANESWAR

Ratikanta Mohapatra is a leading male Odissi dancer. Born into the illustrious family of Guru Kelucharan Mohapatra and Laxmipriya, he has been endowed with all the natural abilities that a dancer should possess. Besides dancing, Ratikanta is a brilliant percussionist of the Odissi *pakhawaj* and a qualified teacher. At present, he is a teacher of Odissi dance and Director of *Srjan*, a premier Odissi institute of our country founded by Guru Kelucharan Mohapatra.

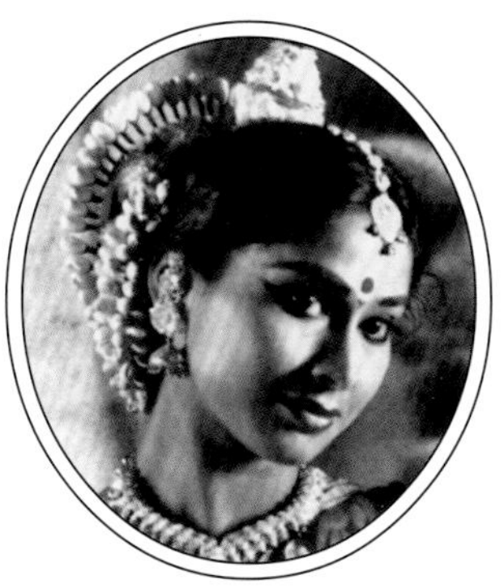

Sujata Mohapatra

BHUBANESWAR

Sujata Mohapatra is a devoted and talented disciple and daughter-in-law of the legendary Guru Kelucharan Mohapatra. She has completed more than 18 years training under the guidance of her Guru. She has also been trained at the Odissi Research Centre at Bhubaneswar.

Sujata has a compelling stage presence and is a rare combination of intensity and spontaneity in dance. Amongst the present generation, she has established herself as a dancer of repute, having achieved the techniques and subtle proportions of the Odissi dance form. She has performed widely in India and abroad.

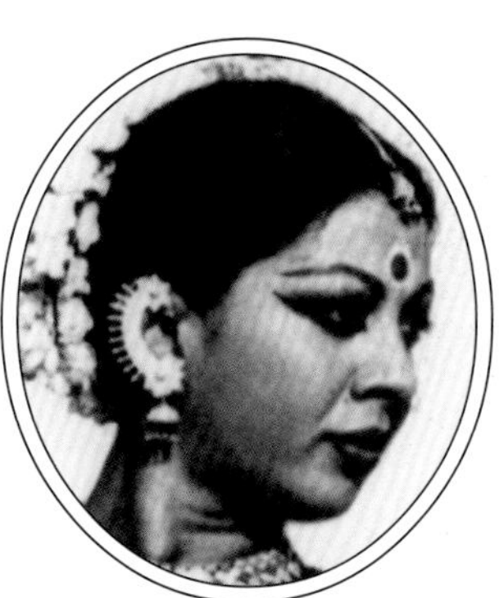

Protima Gauri Bedi

BOMBAY

Initiated into Odissi dance at the age of twenty-six, Protima Gauri Bedi became one of the most well-known dancers in India through sheer grit and will-power. Protima's most notable contribution to the world of Indian classical dance was 'Nrityagram', a dance village situated in the outskirts of Bangalore. 'Nrityagram' was set up for the preservation and popularisation of Odissi and other Indian classical dance styles. She had more than five hundred performances in India and abroad to her credit.

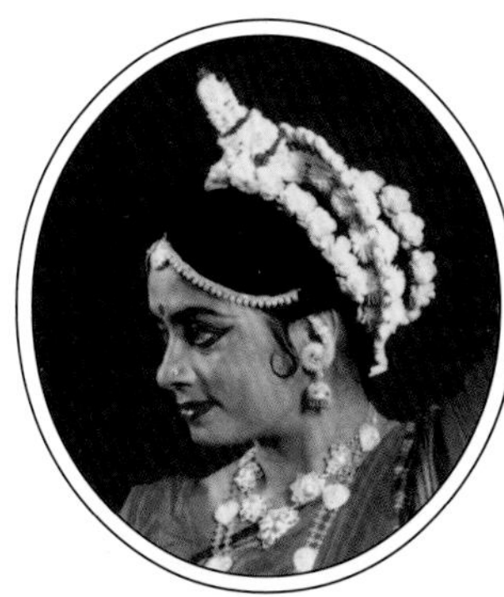

Geeta Mahalik

NOIDA

Geeta Mahalik is a senior disciple of Guru Mayadhar Raut and has given numerous recitals in various festivals in India and abroad. She has composed and choreographed several compositions in Odissi.

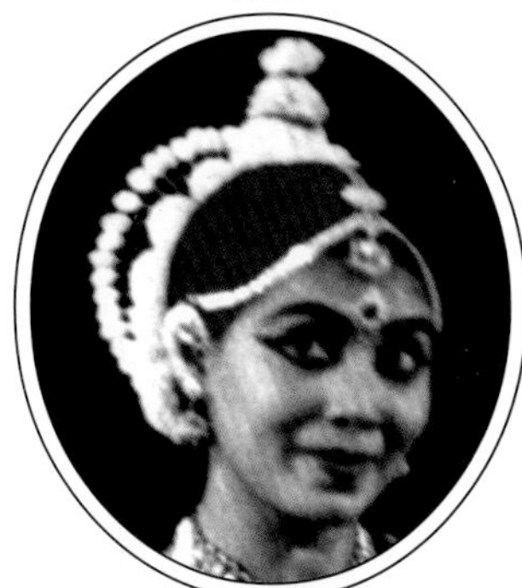

Aruna Mohanty

BHUBANESWAR

Initiated to dance at an early age by Guru Srinath Raut and Guru Govinda Charan Pal, Aruna Mohanty further trained under the eminent Guru Shri Gangadhar Pradhan. She is known for her excellent *abhinaya* and has a natural flair for expressions. She has performed in most of the major cities and festivals within the country and abroad.

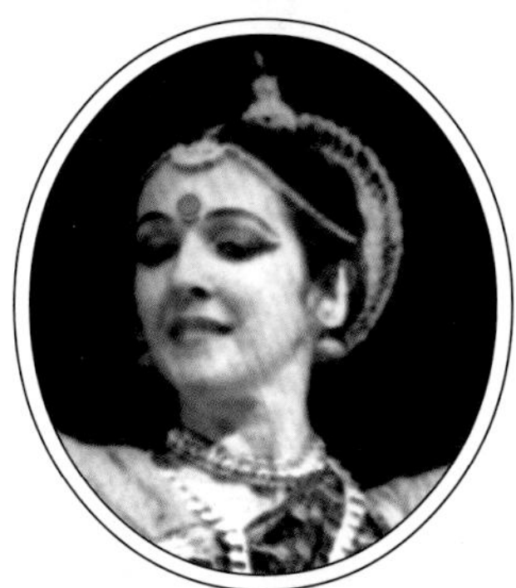

Ileana Citaristi

BHUBANESWAR

Italian by birth, Ileana Citaristi was trained in Odissi dance under Guru Kelucharan Mohapatra. She has learnt the *chhau* dance of Mayurbhanja under the guidance of Guru Shri Hari Nayak. She has done a deep study of Indian culture and philosophy and has received her Ph.D. in Religious Studies from the University of Venice. She is imparting training in Odissi and *chhau* dances to local as well as visiting students in her own institution 'Art Vision' in Bhubaneswar .

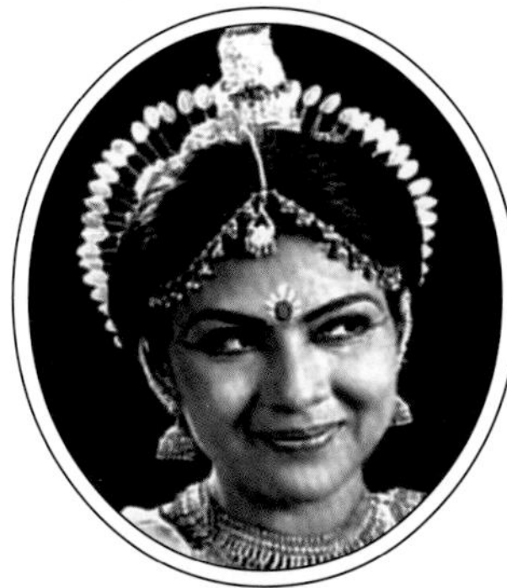

Aloka Kanungo

KOLKATA

Aloka Kanungo is a well-established and multifaceted Odissi dancer who was trained by Guru Raghunath Dutta and Guru Mayadhar Raut, after which she came under the tutelage of the legendary maestro Guru Kelucharan Mohapatra. She has formed 'Shinjan'—a troupe of dedicated students—and has performed at various festivals.

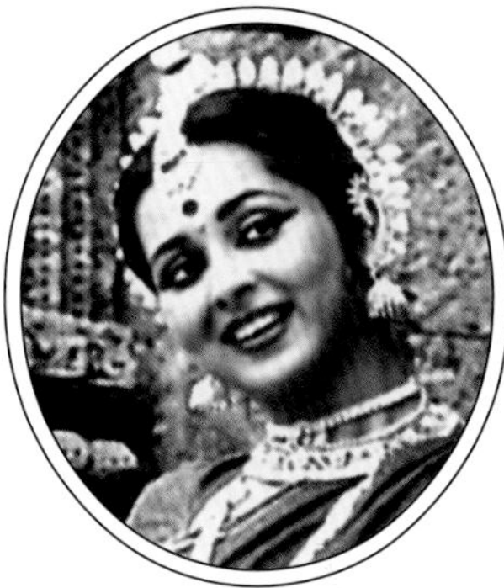

Sharmila Biswas

KOLKATA

Sharmila Biswas received her earlier training from Murlidhar Maji and later under Guru Kelucharan Mohapatra. Through her organisation, 'Odissi Vision and Movement Centre', she has been engaged in teaching and experimenting to enrich the dance and create new choreographic works.

Sangeeta Dash

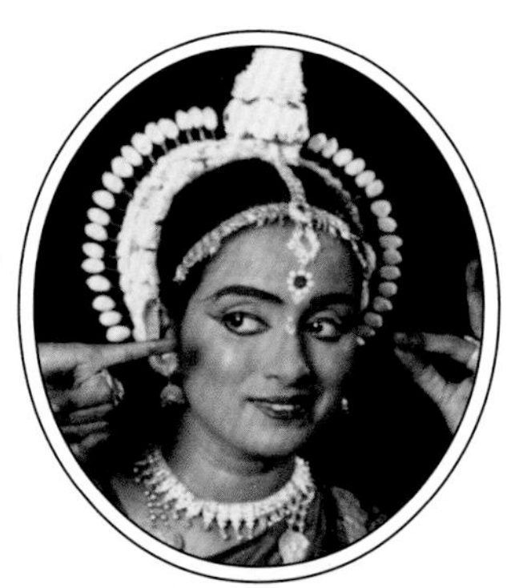

PONDICHERY

Sangeeta Dash started her training at a young age under the guidance of Guru Sri Durga Charan Ranbir and Late Sri Deba Prasad Das until 1986. She is one of the finest amongst the younger generation of Odissi dancers of today and has participated in various dance festivals in India and abroad.

Kavita Dwibedi

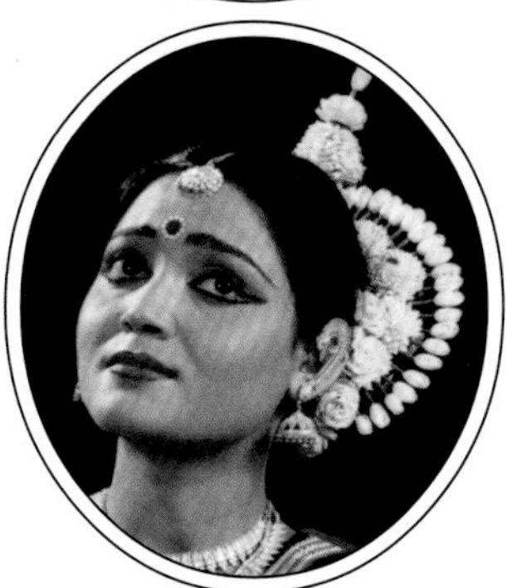

DELHI

Kavita Dwibedi received her training from her father Guru Hare Krishna Behera. She has given performances both in India and abroad. Presently she is working as the founder director of Odissi Akademi, Delhi.

Jyoti Shrivastava

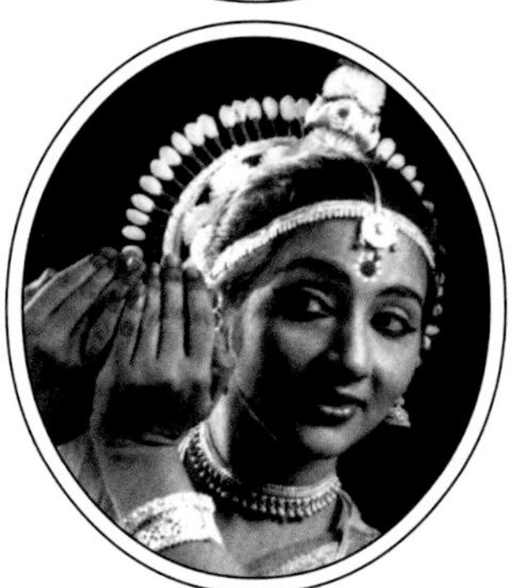

NOIDA

Trained under the late Guru Srinath Raut and later Guru Durga Charan Ranvir, Jyoti Shrivastava has performed extensively and is the recipient of various fellowships and awards. She dedicates her time to perfecting her art and teaching.

Bijayini Satpathy

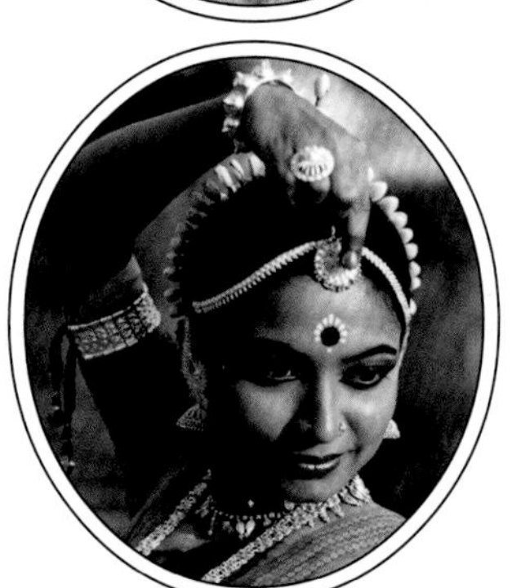

BANGALORE

Bijayini Satpathy began her training at the age of seven under Guru Gangadhar Pradhan and Guru Kanduri Charana Behera. She joined 'Nrityagram' in 1993 under the guidance of Protima Gauri Bedi. At present, she is Director of the Odissi Gurukul at 'Nrityagram' and is involved in the training of a new generation of dancers.

Kasturi Pattanik

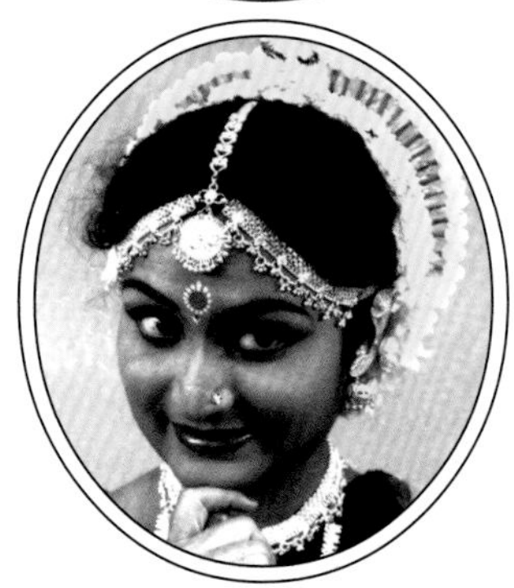

CUTTACK

Kasturi Pattanik has received training at the Odissi Research Centre under the guidance of Guru Kelucharan Mohapatra, Kumkum Mohanty, Sanjukta Panigrahi and Raghunath Dutta. At present she is working as a senior Odissi dance teacher at Odissi Reaserch Centre, Bhubaneswar.

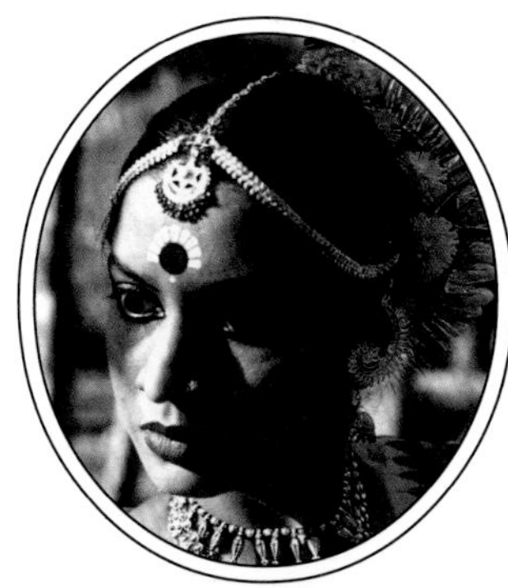

Surupa Sen

BANGALORE

Surupa Sen was trained to be an Odissi dancer by the legendary Guru Kelucharan Mohapatra and Protima Gauri Bedi. At present, she is Creative Director and principal dancer of 'Nrityagram'.

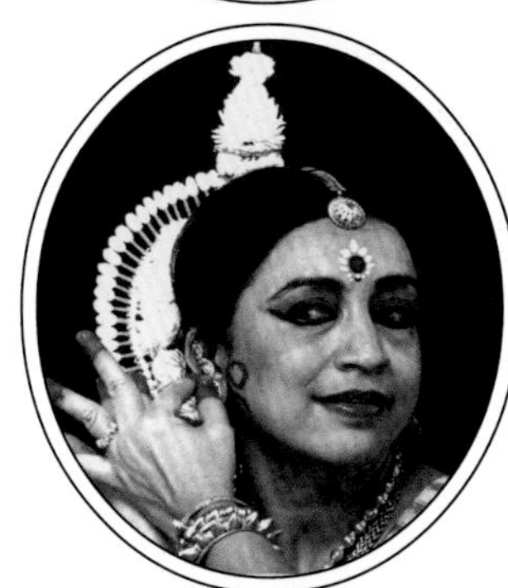

Daksha Mashruwala

MUMBAI

Trained under the distinguished maestro Guru Kelucharan Mohapatra, Daksha Mashruwala is an accomplished Odissi dancer. She has choreographed several compositions and runs a teaching institution, 'Kaishiki'. She has given very successful perfomances in India and abroad.

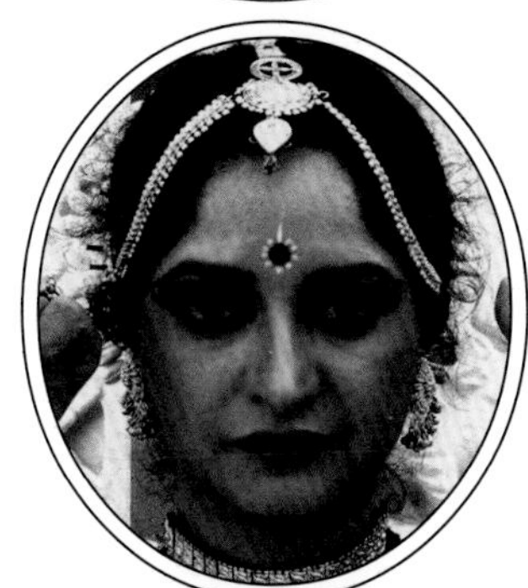

Shagun Butani

DELHI

Shagun Butani commenced her training in Odissi with Aloka Paniker and later trained under Guru Gangadhar Pradhan. She has performed and conducted workshops both within the country and abroad. She is a versatile performer and besides traditional repertoires has done collaborative productions, thus using her experience of the traditional technique in innovative ways.

She has been awarded the Indira Gandhi Priyadarshini Award and is a recipient of a junior fellowship, Ministry of Culture.

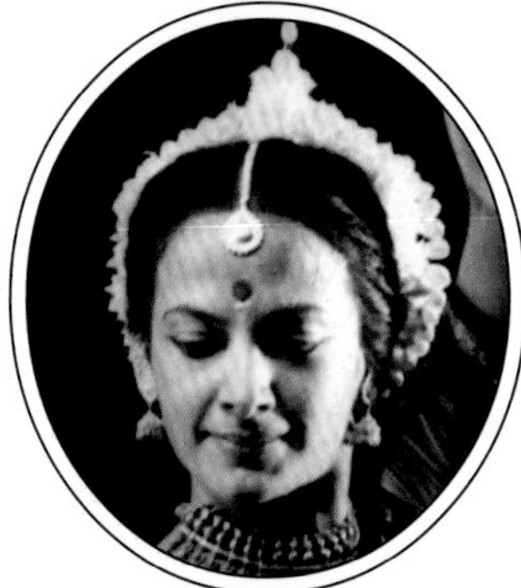

Rekha Tandon

DELHI

Rekha Tandon received her training in Odissi dance Madhvi Mudgal. She also trained under Guru Trinath Maharana. Presently she is working towards a Ph.D. in dance in London. She has won appreciation for her performances. She has made a mark in the field of Odissi dance with her innovative choreography.

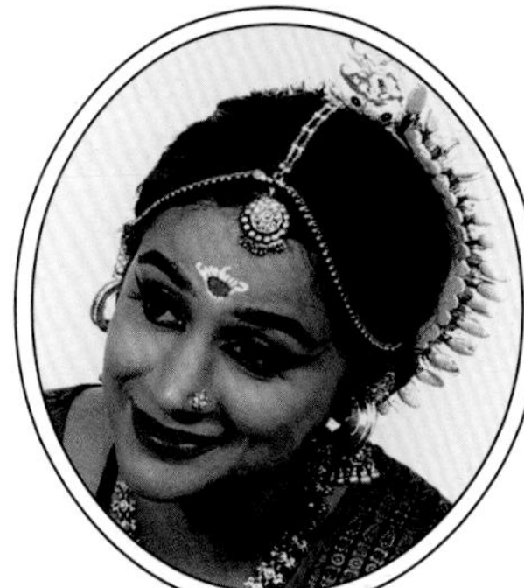

Anandi Ramachandran

MUMBAI

Anandi is a senior disciple of Guru Kelucharan Mohapatra. She has several performances to her credit, both in India and abroad. Apart from dancing, she has acted and choreographed dance pieces in art films.

Glossary

abhinaya	acting
adbhutam	wondrous
aharya	ornaments, make-up, costumes
akhada	training centre for *gotipuas*
alata	red paint for feet and hands
amrit	nectar
angas	body parts
angika	as shown by means of limbs
apsara	celestial dancer
ashtapadi	set of eight *shlokas* from the *Geeta Govinda*
bada sringar	bedtime decoration of Lord Jagannath
bahara gauni	female singer performing outside the inner sanctum
bakula	species of tree
bandha nritya	acrobatic dance performed by *gotipuas*
bengapatia	frog's mouth-shaped waistband or belt
bhakti rasa	expression of devotion
bhangi	stance
bhava	expression or feelings
bhaya	fear
bhitara gauni	female singer inside temple
bhramari	swirling movement in dance; also known as *bhauri*
bhumi	Mother Earth
bhumipranam	salutation to Mother Earth
bibhatsa	disgust
bindi	decorative mark on forehead
chandan	sandalwood paste
chapasari	necklace
char dham	four pilgrimage centres in India: Badrinath, Jagannath, Dwarka, Rameshwaram
chari	dance walk; also known as *chali*
chauk	Odissi dance stance
daitas	tribal priest community of Jagannath Temple

dakshinatya	dance form of South India
dakshini	southern
devadasi	woman dancer in temple service
gandharva	celestial musician
gaudasini	temple servant to fan icons
gopi	milkmaid
gotipua	young male dancer of Odissi
gorachana	sandalwood paste design on forehead and cheeks
hasta	hand
hasta mudra	hand gesture
hasya	humour
jatra	travelling theatre group
kanchula	blouse
kapa	ear ornament
karakankan	wrist ornament
karuna	pathetic
kunchita (pada)	foot position
lasya	feminine dance
laya	pace in rhythm
lokadharmi	folk and traditional elements of performance
madhavika	kind of flower
mahari	temple dancer from Orissa
mangalacharan	first item in the traditional repertoire
mardala	percussion instrument
math	monastery
mina nayak	*mahari's* guard; also *sahi nayak*
moksha	salvation
mukhabhinaya	facial expression
nachuni	dancer; also *nartaki*
natya	play and its production
natyadharmi	production that follows the scriptures
nayaka/nayika	hero/heroine
nibibandha	apron-like cloth with frills to cover hips
nritta	pure dance (technical)
nritya	expressional dance

nupur	ankle bells
pada bheda	foot positions
pada vinaya	foot movement
pakhawaj	percussion instrument
patta	sari border
pushpachuda	kind of hair bun
pushpanjali	flower offering
raga	melody
raj guru	head priest
raslila	group dance by Krishna and his female friends
raudra	furious
sakala dhupa	burning of incense in the morning
sakhi bhava	to feel as Krishna's friend
sakhi nach	to dance as Krishna's friend
sandhya dhupa	burning of incense in the evening
samudra manthan	churning of the ocean
sarga	chapter
sattvika	pure
seva	service
shanta	peace
shastra	scripture
shloka	Sanskrit couplet
shringara	amorous
shringara bhakti	devotion portrayed through eroticism / love
shringara rasa	one of nine *rasas* described in the scriptures
stupa	in this case, pillar
tala	time-cycle beat
tandav	masculine
tamala	species of tree
tayita	armlet
tribhangi	three-bend body stance in Odissi
trikhandi pranam	series of three salutations: to the gods; to the guru; to the audience
ukuta	small unit of syllables
utha, baitha,	

thia, chali burha, bhasa, bhauri, pali	Odissi dance positions
vachika	spoken/sound
veenakara	player of the *veena,* a musical instrument
veera	brave
vritti	characteristics
yogini	ascetic woman

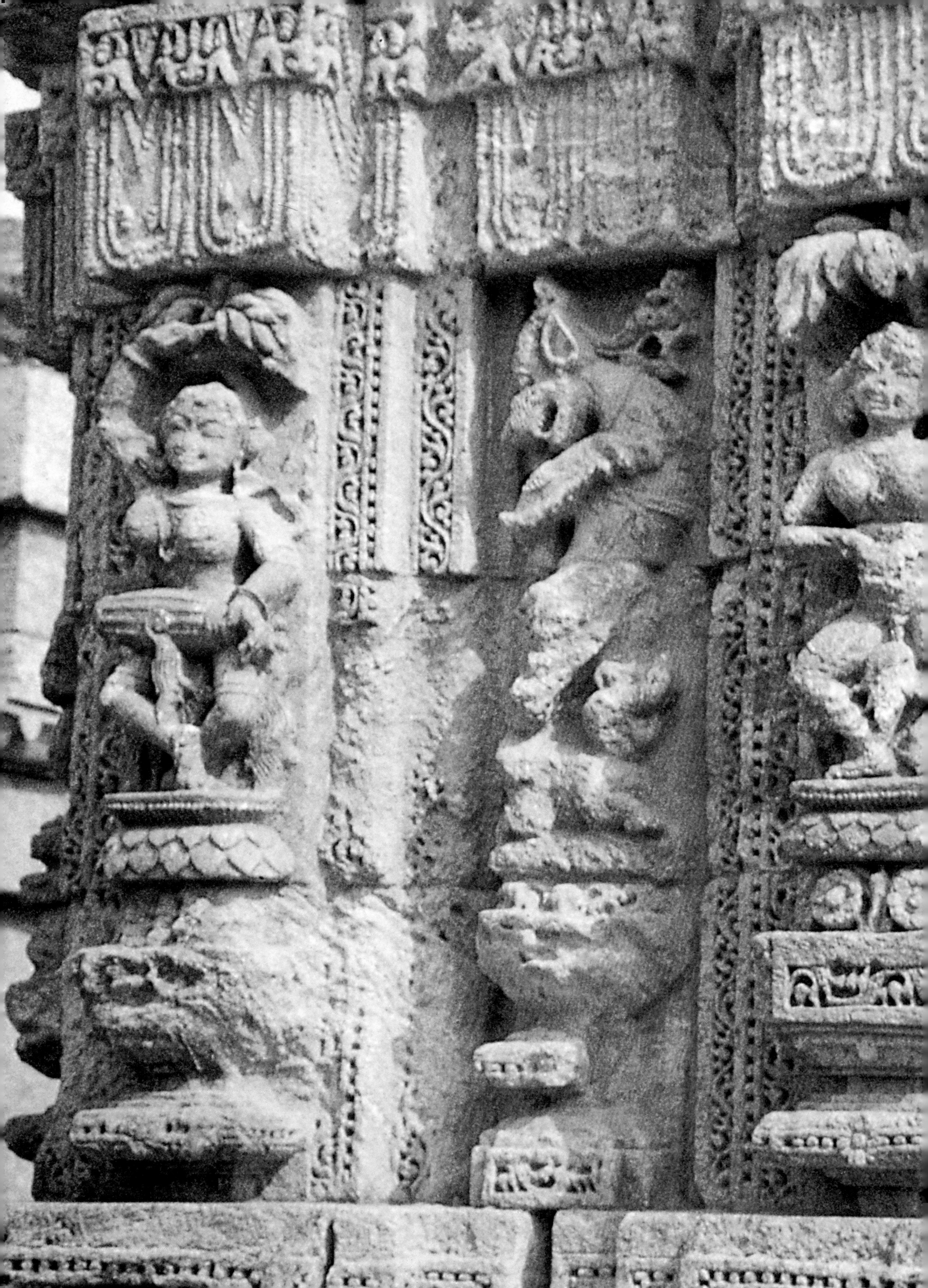